W9-AFS-470

Defusing Disruptive Behavior

A Workbook for Health Care Leaders

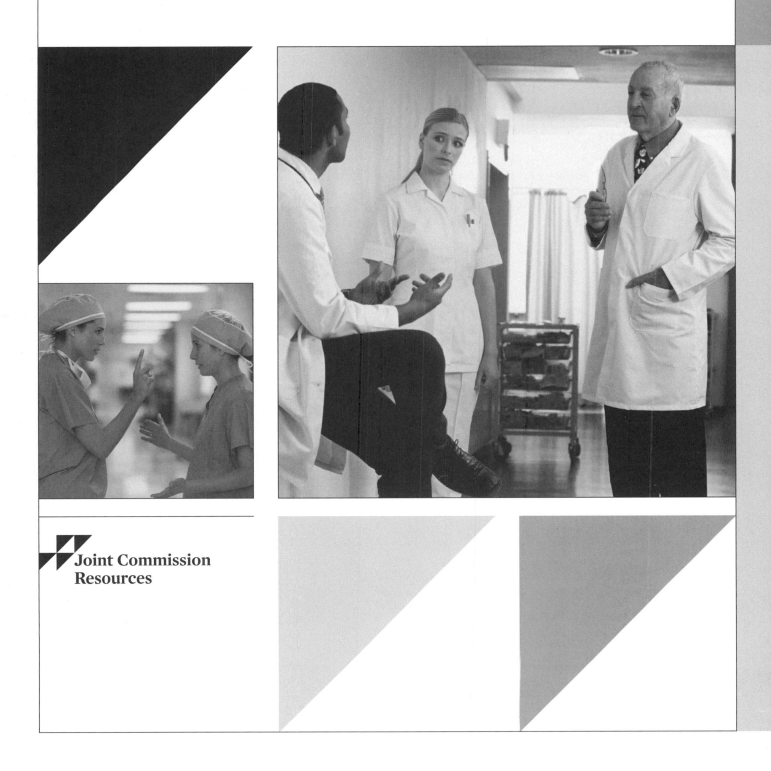

Joint Commission Resources

Senior Editor: Audrie Armes
Project Manager: Andrew Bernotas
Manager, Publications: Paul Reis
Associate Director, Production: Johanna Harris
Associate Director: Cecily Pew
Executive Director: Catherine Chopp Hinckley
Vice President, Learning: Charles Macfarlane, F.A.C.H.E.
Joint Commission/JCR Reviewers: Pat Adamski, Peter Angood, M.D., Darlene Christiansen, Hal Bressler, Thomas Wallace, M.D.

Joint Commission Resources Mission

The mission of Joint Commission Resources is to continuously improve the safety and quality of care in the United States and in the international community through the provision of education and consultation services and international accreditation.

Joint Commission Resources educational programs and publications support, but are separate from, the accreditation activities of The Joint Commission. Attendees at Joint Commission Resources educational programs and purchasers of Joint Commission Resources publications receive no special consideration or treatment in, or confidential information about, the accreditation process.

The inclusion of an organization name, product, or service in a Joint Commission publication should not be construed as an endorsement of such organization, product, or services, nor is failure to include an organization name, product, or service to be construed as disapproval.

This publication is designed to provide accurate and authoritative information in regard to the subject matter covered. Every attempt has been made to ensure accuracy at the time of publication; however, please note that laws, regulations, and standards are subject to change. Please also note that some of the examples in this publication are specific to the laws and regulations of the locality of the facility. The information and examples in this publication are provided with the understanding that the publisher is not engaged in providing medical, legal, or other professional advice. If any such assistance is desired, the services of a competent professional person should be sought.

© 2007 by the Joint Commission on Accreditation of Healthcare Organizations

Joint Commission Resources, Inc. (JCR), a not-for-profit affiliate of The Joint Commission, has been designated by The Joint Commission to publish publications and multimedia products. JCR reproduces and distributes these materials under license from The Joint Commission.

All rights reserved. No part of this publication may be reproduced in any form or by any means without written permission from the publisher.

Printed in the U.S.A. 5 4 3 2 1

Requests for permission to make copies of any part of this work should be mailed to:
Permissions Editor
Department of Publications
Joint Commission Resources
One Renaissance Boulevard
Oakbrook Terrace, Illinois 60181
permissions@jcrinc.com

ISBN: 978-1-59940-084-6
Library of Congress Control Number: 2007929874

For more information about Joint Commission Resources, please visit http://www.jcrinc.com.

Contents

Disruptive Behavior and Its Impact on the Culture of Safety

The importance of culture in creating a safe environment has long been recognized, as evidenced by the widespread use of the term *culture of safety*. Industries that have succeeded in vastly reducing accident rates and achieving highly reliable performance, such as aviation and nuclear power, have done so in great part because they have embraced the elements of a culture of safety. These elements include a nonpunitive approach to error, a flattened hierarchy that encourages input from all team members—regardless of rank—on areas within their expertise, and empowerment of all team members to speak up if they perceive a threat to safety. A culture of safety is characterized by a collective mindfulness that can be achieved only when there is mutual respect among team members and an absence of fear and intimidation.

Although patient safety has received much attention since the Institute of Medicine's 1999 report on medical errors,[1] progress in achieving a culture of safety in health care organizations is less certain. According to data released by the Agency for Healthcare Research and Quality (AHRQ), only 70% of hospital workers surveyed agreed that management's actions show that patient safety is a top priority. In the same survey, only 75% of respondents agreed that staff members freely speak up if they see something that may negatively affect patient care, and only 46% reported feeling free to question the decisions or actions of those with more authority. A full 62% of respondents reported that they are afraid to ask questions when things don't seem quite right.[2]

Clearly, authority gradient and intimidation remain powerful forces in health care organizations. Diametrically opposed as they are to the principles of a culture of safety, they stand in the way of true progress on patient safety. Perhaps one of the most disturbing signs of this lack of progress in fostering a culture of safety is the prevalence of disruptive clinician behavior, which has long been tolerated by health care organizations

unwilling to confront the problem. Indeed, more than 95% of physician executives who responded to an American College of Physician Executives survey reported encountering disturbing, disruptive, and potentially dangerous behaviors on a regular basis.[3] Likewise, in a 2002 survey of Veterans Health Administration hospitals, 96% of nurses reported witnessing or experiencing disruptive physician behavior.[4] Physicians were not the only offenders, with nurses, pharmacists, and radiology and laboratory staff also identified as being disruptive in other survey research.[5,6]

The Impact of Disruptive Behavior

The impact of disruptive behavior on patient safety has been well described in the literature. Intimidation is the goal and frequent outcome of such behavior, with those on the receiving end often acquiescing to a disrupter's unreasonable demands, even when the safety of the patient may be at risk.[6] Employee morale and nurse turnover also suffer as a result of disruptive behavior.[5,7,8] There are other costs as well, including those associated with rework, lost productivity, and managing staff emotional turmoil and stress that distract attention and resources from providing safe patient care.

Despite the risks and costs of disruptive behavior, health care organizations are often reluctant to confront the problem, particularly when it involves physicians. Those responsible for addressing the behavior find it to be a difficult and unpleasant task, and even when they do so, organizational mechanisms often prove inadequate to solve the problem.[3,5,9–12] As a result, such behavior frequently persists over long periods of time and becomes the norm.

There is mounting evidence to suggest that this "hands-off" approach by health care leaders will no longer be tolerated, particularly by staff on the receiving end of the behavior. Consider the following accounts from the news media:

Highland Surgeon Suspended, May Be Charged:
Drunken Altercation Reported in Hospital's Operating
Room
San Francisco Chronicle, March 9, 2006

Doctor Must Pay in Bullying Case
Indianapolis Star, March 5, 2005

In both instances, staff grew tired of dealing with bullying behavior by physicians and resorted to the legal system to redress their grievances. One case resulted in criminal charges against the offending physician, while the other resulted in a jury verdict against the physician after a civil suit was filed by a hospital staff member. In both instances, the organizations at which these incidents occurred endured protracted negative media attention and loss of reputation as a result.

There are signs that The Joint Commission, health care's largest and most influential accrediting organization, has also tired of health care organizations' lax treatment of this problem. Standards approved by the Board of Commissioners address the responsibility of leaders to monitor organizational culture and deal with cultural problems, including disruptive behavior. Furthermore, the Joint Commission's Sentinel Event Advisory Group has also recognized the importance of this issue and has released a potential National Patient Safety Goal for field review, though it has not yet adopted such a goal.

There are liability exposures associated with disruptive behavior as well, although they have not been fully explored in the literature. These include potential claims of hostile work environment brought by employees and contract staff, workers' compensation claims for workplace stress, directors' and officers' claims against organizations that fail to monitor the problem or take action against reported offenders by continuing to renew employment or privileges, general liability claims brought by visitors and other bystanders injured as a result of disruptive behavior, and medical malpractice claims brought by patients injured as a result of a clinician's disruptive behavior.

Many compelling reasons can be found for organizations to confront the problem of disruptive behavior and adopt a zero-tolerance approach. Health care organizations are already suffering from staffing shortages and are challenged by employee morale issues, as demonstrated by the AHRQ survey.

Avoidance of adverse publicity and financial loss from liability and other claims is also potent a motivator because it supports the imperative of continued financial viability and organizational survival.

Although all these are compelling arguments, none are as important as the human considerations—the devastating impact that disruptive behavior has on the dignity, self-esteem, and physical safety of staff members and patients alike.

Change and the desire for it should come not because of disruptive behavior's impact on morale, staff turnover, or liability. Rather, change should be motivated by the recognition that this behavior is simply incompatible with the core values of health care professionals and the organizations they work in, and it is at odds with that all-important phrase first uttered so long ago and more recently invoked by the Institute of Medicine—"first, do no harm."

Defusing Disruptive Behavior: A Workbook for Health Care Leaders is one step toward this change and toward creating a true culture of safety in health care.

Grena Porto, R.N., M.S., A.R.M., C.P.H.R.M., *Senior vice president, Marsh, Inc., Philadelphia, and member of The Joint Commission's Sentinel Event Advisory Group.*

References

1. Kohn L.T., et al. (eds.): *To Err Is Human: Building a Safer Health System.* Washington, DC: National Academy Press, 1999.
2. Agency for Healthcare Research and Quality: *Hospital Survey on Patient Safety Culture: 2007 Comparative Database Report,* Apr. 2007. http://www.ahrq.gov/qual/hospsurveydb/ (accessed Jul. 9, 2007).
3. Weber D.O.: Poll results: Doctors' disruptive behavior disturbs physician leaders. *Physician Exec* 30(4):6–14, 2004.
4. Rosenstein A.H.: Nurse–physician relationships: Impact on nurse satisfaction and retention. *Am J Nurs* 102(6):26–34, 2002.
5. Rosenstein A.H., O'Daniel M.: Disruptive behavior and clinical outcomes: Perceptions of nurses and physicians. *Am J Nurs* 105(1):54–64, 2005.
6. Institute for Safe Medication Practices: *Results from ISMP Survey on Workplace Intimidation,* 2003. http://www.ismp.org/Survey/surveyresults/Survey0311.asp (accessed Jul. 9, 2007).
7. Diaz A.L., McMillin J.D.: A definition and description of nurse abuse. *West J Nurs Res* 3(1):97–109, 1991.
8. Cox H.C.: Verbal abuse in nursing: Report of a study. *Nurs Manag* 18:47–50, 1987.

9. Leape L.L., Fromson J.A.: Problem doctors: Is there a system-level solution? *Ann Intern Med* 144(2):107–115, 2006.
10. Linney B.J.: Confronting the disruptive physician. *Physician Exec* 23:55–58, 1997.
11. Benzer D.G., Miller M.M.: The disruptive-abusive physician: A new look at an old problem. *WMJ* 94:455–460, 1995.
12. Neff, K.E.: Understanding and managing physicians with disruptive behavior. In Ransom S.B., Pinsky W.W., Tropman J.E. (eds.): *Enhancing Physician Performance: Advanced Principles of Medical Management.* Tampa, FL: American College of Healthcare Executives, 2000, pp. 45–72.

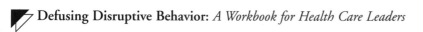

Introduction

Health care in the twenty-first century is experiencing the growing pains of evolution. There have been a number of contributing factors, but when the Institute of Medicine published its seminal work *To Err Is Human* in 1999, a broad, far-sweeping shift in mind-set began among health care organizations. Although the industry had already been discussing the imperative for a systems-based focus on improving the quality and safety of care, treatment, and services, the entire field was now faced with a disturbing fact: Certain unsafe and unacceptable practices that had become the norm in many health care organizations were causing medical errors resulting in serious injury and death. This broader awareness led to a sense of urgency to improve patient safety and prevent such dire outcomes.

As a result, health care organizations and national accrediting bodies have sharpened their focus on patient safety. The Joint Commission, which has been drawing attention to patient safety and quality issues since its inception, has been a leader in this effort with its standards and National Patient Safety Goals. Its revamped accreditation process—launched in 2004—uses new methodologies to help organizations see how their systems of providing safe, high-quality care, treatment, and services are functioning. This sharpened focus includes not only the call to strengthen efforts to avoid adverse events in health care but also to establish and maintain a culture of safety, thus ensuring that organizations would truly achieve their goal of being patient safety focused. (In 2007, new medical staff standards now consider "professionalism" as part of competency, which includes ethics and disruptive behavior. This is another step in the process.)

A Culture of Safety

In a health care organization a *culture of safety* promotes, embraces, and applies consistent patient safety principles. Organization policies and procedures that require safe prac-

tices are only part of the story—in a culture of safety, staff will demand safety and have no tolerance for unsafe practices. The Institute for Healthcare Improvement describes a culture of safety as an environment in which "people are not merely encouraged to work toward change; they take action when it is needed. Inaction in the face of safety problems is taboo, and eventually the pressure comes from all directions—from peers as well as leaders. There is no room in a culture of safety for those who uselessly point fingers or say, 'Safety is not my responsibility, so I'll file a report and wash my hands of it.'"[1]

Establishing a culture of safety is akin to following the Golden Rule. "Do unto others as you would have done to you" is a principle that can and should apply in the health care work environment. Everyone wants to be respected, and all people want their contributions to make a difference. In a culture of safety, the organization fosters an environment in which all staff members are respected, empowered, and focused on the noble nature of their profession: providing for the health and well-being of the populations they serve.

But establishing a culture of safety is no simple task. There is no magic wand that will miraculously implement one in a health care organization. Organizations have found that although some elements are relatively straightforward to adopt—appointing and establishing a patient safety committee, for example—others take more time and effort. The "culture" part of the equation requires a change in mind-set, and the change has to be embraced organizationwide—from board members to support staff. Changing the organization mind-set requires examining cultural habits that have adversely affected patient safety (for example, poor communication or inadequate teamwork). Many organizations have found that one such detrimental cultural habit is the toleration of disruptive behavior.

Disruptive Behavior

Disruptive behavior has been defined by the Joint Commission as "conduct by a health care professional that intimidates others working in the organization to the extent that quality and safety are compromised." Research has found that disruptive behavior not only impacts the morale and staffing of an organization but can also lead to medical errors and breakdowns in the quality of care, treatment, and services delivered. Disruptive behavior—and its potentially dire outcomes—runs contrary to the concept of a culture of safety. Addressing such behavior in the health care workplace is therefore essential. The Joint Commission now expects all accredited health care organizations to adopt processes and procedures to effectively deal with disruptive behavior. This expectation is illustrated by the publication of new elements of performance under Standard LD.3.10—the standard that requires organizations to establish a culture of safety and quality.*

Navigating the Work Environment

The work environment isn't always a straightforward place to navigate, as anyone who has spent a day on any job can attest. The complexity and variability of the work environment can be challenging and stressful. Sometimes the stress comes from the job itself, and sometimes it comes from conditions in the environment or disputes with coworkers. Each person brings different talents, competencies, and abilities to the job, and these individual skills enable each staff member to add something unique to the position. But workplace conflict can sometimes erupt. Such a complex environment has the potential for problems, and that complexity can create a perfect storm of ups and downs.

Disruptive Behavior in the Workplace

From harassment and intimidation to abuse and assault, disruptive behavior in the workplace has a devastating impact on morale and productivity. Health care is not immune to such behavior. In fact, many health care organizations seem to tolerate staff members' rudeness, intimidation, insults, threats, passive-aggressive behavior, verbal abuse, and even physical assault (or the threat thereof). Victims are expected to "get used to it," particularly when the perpetrator is a physician. Of course, nurses, pharmacists, technicians, administrators, and other staff are also capable of exhibiting disruptive behavior—no area of health care has been left untouched by its impact.

When organization leaders tolerate disruptive behavior, the results can include lower morale, higher turnover, and reduced patient safety. In such a "toxic environment," staff members might also begin to demonstrate additional negative behaviors, such as poor communication, hostility, resentment, stress, anxiety, avoidance, or fear—all of which impair an organization's ability to deliver safe, high-quality patient care.

About This Publication

Defusing Disruptive Behavior: A Workbook for Health Care Leaders provides the background, information, and tools that leaders need to establish effective policies and procedures for dealing with disruptive behavior. In addition to methods of defusing disruptive behavior, proactive procedures such as conflict resolution are discussed. The publication also includes extensive scenarios, helpful case studies, sample policies from organizations around the country, discussion points, and forms and worksheets. Discussion questions have been interspersed throughout the text to give readers a chance to reflect on the content and how it relates to the unique issues in their own organizations. In addition, several sidebars feature health care leaders sharing their personal experiences and advice about disruptive behavior.

Terms Used in This Publication

Across the broad spectrum of health care organizations, different terms are sometimes used to refer to individuals who receive care, treatment, and services. For the sake of simplicity and clarity, the term *patient* is used in this publication to refer to those individuals. The term *health care organization* is used to refer to organizations that provide care, treatment, and services, except when an example refers to a specific kind of health care organization.

Acknowledgments

The process of developing a book often involves the significant help and contributions of many individuals to help shape the content. This book is no exception. Joint Commission Resources (JCR) would therefore like to thank the following individuals for their invaluable insight and perspective: Thomas Wallace, M.D., J.D., M.B.A.; John-Henry Pfifferling, Ph.D.; Ron May, M.D.; Lawrence Shuer, M.D.; Rick Croteau, M.D.; Bill Swiggart, M.A.; Mike Cohen, Pharm.D.; and

---

* These new requirements are effective January 1, 2009.

Nancee Bender, Ph.D., R.N. A particular note of thanks is offered to Grena Porto, R.N., M.S.N., for writing the foreword. JCR also wishes to thank the many reviewers who have lent their expert eye to the development of the content and Ladan Cockshut for her hard work and dedication in writing this book.

Reference

1. Institute for Healthcare Improvement: *Develop a Culture of Safety.* http://www.ihi.org/IHI/Topics/PatientSafety/SafetyGeneral/Changes/ Develop+a+Culture+of+Safety.htm (accessed Jun. 1, 2007).

Defusing Disruptive Behavior: *A Workbook for Health Care Leaders*

Chapter 1

Defining Disruptive Behavior

In this chapter: This chapter describes and defines disruptive behavior and provides examples. It discusses why some health care workers might behave in this manner and what happens to morale, communication, and job functions when disruptive behavior impedes safe patient care. The chapter also profiles the forthcoming elements of performance related to disruptive behavior that appear in Standard LD.3.10—the "culture of safety" standard.

The camera zooms in on the Hollywood actor playing the role of the archetypal surgeon as he reviews the chart of a patient who looks in need of a medical miracle. Beside the surgeon is a female resident who has been overseeing the care of the patient. As she begins to provide information about the patient, the surgeon brushes her off with a wave and barks orders to a nurse standing nearby. When the nurse begins to ask a question regarding one of the orders, the surgeon abruptly cuts her off. The nurse is taken aback by the surgeon's harsh tone but handles the orders.

As the scene continues and the tension mounts, the surgeon's behavior becomes even more abrupt as he struggles to complete his near-impossible task. But with his exceptional skill, he overcomes the odds, the patient survives, and the surgeon is hailed as a miracle worker by the end of the episode.

Such scenes are common on television medical dramas, and the stereotypes they perpetuate—the intimidated resident, the overbearing surgeon, and the bullied nurse (with the patient stuck somewhere in the middle, hoping for a miracle)—may promote the perception of disruptive behavior in the health care workplace as the norm. From the perspective of the layperson viewing the show, such behavior may therefore seem

acceptable (or at least inevitable). But as anyone who has experienced disruptive behavior in any work environment knows, this behavior should not be accepted and never needs to be viewed as inevitable. The effects of disruptive behavior are detrimental to staff morale and, in the case of health care organizations, may contribute to adverse outcomes for patients. Working to defuse and prevent disruptive behavior should be the goal of all health care organizations as part of an overall strategy to establish and sustain a culture of safety.

Although behavior such as that exhibited by the fictional surgeon described here may make for entertaining television, it interferes with the proper functioning of a health care organization. Disruptive behavior can hinder effective teamwork; reduce staff satisfaction, which can lead to burnout and a high turnover rate; impair organization morale; and negatively affect the organization's bottom line.[1] But the damage caused by disruptive behavior isn't limited to human resources and financial issues. The most devastating effect of such behavior in a health care organization is its potential impact on patient safety.

What Is Disruptive Behavior?

The term *disruptive behavior* has been defined by The Joint Commission as follows:

Conduct by an individual working in the organization that intimidates others to the extent that quality and safety are compromised. Organizations will define disruptive and inappropriate behaviors for themselves, but in general these behaviors may be verbal or nonverbal and may involve the use of rude language, may be threatening, and may even involve physical contact. Anyone who works in the organization can display disruptive and inappropriate behaviors, including management, clinical and administrative staff, licensed independent practitioners, and governing body members.

Essentially, then, any behavior that interferes with the ability of others to effectively carry out their duties or that undermines a patient's confidence in the organization or another member of the health care team can be considered disruptive.[2] In addition, some actions that might not be considered disruptive when observed as isolated incidents could be classified as disruptive if they are repeated over time and thus form a pattern of inappropriate conduct. Examples of disruptive behavior include the following[2]:

• Profane or disrespectful language
• Demeaning behavior, such as name-calling
• Sexual comments or innuendo
• Inappropriate touching, sexual or otherwise
• Racial or ethnic jokes
• Outbursts of anger
• Throwing of instruments, charts, or other objects
• Criticism of other caregivers in front of patients or other staff
• Comments that undermine a caregiver's self-confidence in caring for patients
• Failure to adequately address safety concerns or patient care needs expressed by another caregiver
• Intimidating behavior that has the effect of suppressing input by other members of the health care team
• Retaliation against any member of the health care team who has reported an instance of violation of the organization's established code of conduct or who has participated in the investigation of such an incident, regardless of the perceived veracity of the report

John-Henry Pfifferling, Ph.D., director of the Center for Professional Well-Being, based in Durham, North Carolina, describes disruptive behavior as "Actions that are experienced as anger, intimidation, and the threat of harm. Substantiated acts of disruptive behavior are at the least uncivil, and at the worst criminal."[1] He goes on to stress that disruptive behavior harms collaborative care and collegiality and that it promotes an abusive and "toxic" workplace.

It is important to note that if a health care worker's ability to function effectively is impaired by substance abuse or certain medical or psychiatric conditions, this is also considered disruptive behavior. Because impairment issues involve a staff member's health, the organization should have policies in place to deal with them. Thomas Wallace, M.D., J.D., M.B.A., experienced chief medical officer and consultant for Joint Commission Resources, notes that an impaired clinician's disruptive behavior could result in adverse outcomes for patients. He has compiled a list of signs to help identify impairment in physicians (*see* Sidebar 1-1, right).

Sidebar 1-1
Signs of an Impaired Physician

Physical Appearance
• Personality or behavior changes
• Deterioration of hygiene or appearance
• Frequent or unusual accidents
• Multiple prescriptions

In the Office
• Frequent or unexplained absences
• Complains of excessive workload
• Inaccessible ("locked door syndrome")
• Excessive ordering of drugs or excessive personal drug use
• Complaints by patients or staff

In the Hospital
• Frequent trips to the restroom
• Frequently late, absent, or ill
• Desire to work alone or refusing work relief
• Lack of or inappropriate responses to pages or calls
• Decreasing quality of performance or patient care

In the Community
• Unreliability or neglect of commitments
• Isolation or withdrawal
• Unpredictable behavior
• Embarrassing behavior at social functions
• Arrest for DUI or other legal problems

Source: Thomas Wallace, M.D., J.D., M.B.A. Used with permission.

The American Medical Association (AMA) defines disruptive behavior by physicians as follows:

A style of interaction with physicians, hospital personnel, patients, family members, or others that interferes with patient care. Such behavior may be expressed verbally by using foul or threatening language, or through non-verbal behavior such as personal habits, for example facial expressions or manners. It may affect the broader operations of an institution, or relate more narrowly to one's ability to work with others, such as unwillingness to work with or inability to relate to other staff in ways that affect patient care. In addition, it may have negative effects on the learning environment of an educational institution—by modeling inappropriate behaviors for students and residents, and by impairing their ability to achieve clinical skills.

Behavior that tends to cause distress among other staff and affect overall morale within the work environment, undermining productivity and possibly leading to high staff turnover or even resulting in ineffective or substandard care would fall within the definition of disruptive behavior. However, criticism that is offered in good faith with the aim of improving patient care should not be construed as disruptive behavior.

In some instances, disruptive behavior may be the manifestation of an underlying condition that requires special attention. Disruptive behavior, such as aggressiveness, intrusiveness, and hyperactivity, or irritability and argumentativeness can be the effects of stress, substance abuse or withdrawal, or dementia. Also of concern are other psychiatric illnesses or organic disorders that affect physicians in ways that cause disruption within the medical care environment.[3]

While the AMA definition applies to physicians specifically, the concepts contained within it can relate to disruptive behavior perpetrated by any staff member in a health care organization.

Emergence of Disruptive Behavior in Health Care

Disruptive behavior in health care is not a new phenomenon. The historical work climate in health care—with its hierarchical roles and largely gender-dominated positions that seemed to promote a subservient/authoritative interaction—often provided favorable conditions for disruptive behavior. Even in recent memory, it was widely accepted that certain positions in a health care organization—such as a physician in a hospital—had a privileged status that allowed great latitude in staff interaction. This would lead, at times, to disruptive behavior that included verbal or physical abuse, disrespect of other staff members, harassment, and inappropriate language. Within such a climate, the individual's oversight of care was viewed as more important than a team approach. With some individuals, that

responsibility—the oversight of care—meant that their perspective on how it should be carried out was superior and the only one that mattered. Questioning the clinician was not acceptable. Unfortunately, this attitude often led to disruptive behavior. Those who had to interact with this type of staff member learned to deal with the disruptive behavior as part of their regular duties. Having to endure such conduct would become a "rite of passage" for new staff. And reporting the actions of a disruptive staff member was often met with indifference and, sometimes, punitive retaliation. Often, the complaint would simply be filed away, and the complainant would receive a seemingly sympathetic response, but he or she would be instructed to accept and "deal with" the situation; for the victim of disruptive behavior, the only choices seemed to be to accept it or leave the organization.

Disruptive behavior often produced more disruptive behavior. New staff, being trained by senior staff members, observed the way their mentors treated other staff and mentally (often subconsciously) took note. Disruptive behavior would thus spread through all levels of staff and come to be considered the norm in the workplace.

In recent years, however, concepts such as the healthy work environment,* human factors engineering, and interdisciplinary teamwork have emerged as important components of an effective patient safety–oriented work environment. Patient safety experts have been carefully examining staff interactions in health care organizations and have begun to correlate disruptive behavior with an increased chance for adverse outcomes. Research demonstrating the effects of such conduct has strengthened the resolve of leaders to establish a culture of safety in their organizations, including the creation of policies for dealing with disruptive behavior. They now recognize that simply enduring disruptive behavior is unacceptable and that the previous mindset that tolerated it must change.

Organizational Impact on Disruptive Behavior

For the most part, perpetrators of disruptive behavior are individual staff members in an organization and represent isolated events, but an organization itself can have an impact on the climate of disruptive behavior. If an organization and its leaders do not promote a climate where the behavior is addressed and consistent steps are put in place to defuse or prevent disruptive behavior from happening, they could be seen as supporting (or at

---

* For more information on healthy work environments, go to
  http://www.aacn.org. Also see Chapter 5, page 89, and the Appendix.

least being apathetic toward) disruptive behavior. One example of such a potentially demoralizing atmosphere would be an organization that openly tolerates the disruptive behavior of a few elite staff members because they are highly effective revenue generators. Other staff in that environment may well begin to exhibit the same type of undesirable behaviors and contribute to a growing toxic work environment. Disruptive behavior that is not addressed will fester and continue to grow in the organization, sapping the resources and time of the administration, staff, and medical staff. This will result in large costs, both financially and in human time and capital, to the organization. Not addressing the behavior directly is not an option.

In addition, when the work environment itself is not striving toward a culture of safety and is thereby not addressing the various factors that need to be in place to ensure its successful establishment, it will not be able to move beyond disruptive behavior. The most effective way to ensure that disruptive behavior does not take place in an organization is for the organization itself to move beyond a culture of disruptive behavior. Leaders must, therefore, take a strong and unmistakable position against disruptive behavior and incorporate proactive measures to defuse and prevent its perpetration. Subsequent chapters in this book discuss ways that organizations can accomplish this. The "For Your Consideration" on page 15 provides questions that leaders can ask themselves to determine whether their organization has an environment that is tolerant of disruptive behavior.

Prevalence of Disruptive Behavior in Health Care Organizations: A Systemic Problem

Although disruptive behavior was more prevalent in the past than it is today and there has been a reduction in such behavior among newer generations of health care professionals, research shows that it still exists and is a serious problem in many organizations. The research also indicates that disruptive behavior can take several forms and affects both staff and patients.[4] For example, recent studies show that the vast majority of staff in hospitals and other health care organizations still find themselves on the receiving end of disruptive behavior and that this conduct is not limited to one particular profession.*

A 2003 study by the Institute for Safe Medication Practices (ISMP) found that 88% of 2,095 survey respondents had experienced disruptive behavior. The respondents reported

having experienced condescending language (88%, with 21% describing it as "often"), impatience with questions (79%; 19% "often"), and reluctance or refusal to answer questions or phone calls (79%; 14% "often"). Even more startling was the reported incidence of abuse, with 48% of respondents stating that they have been subjected to strong verbal abuse, 43% reporting threatening body language, and 4% reporting physical abuse. For many respondents, experiencing disruptive behavior was not an isolated incident with just one staff member. In fact, 38% of respondents reported experiencing disruptive behavior from three to five individuals. It is important to note that the disruptive behavior reported by most respondents was not limited to physicians or other licensed independent practitioners.[5]

In a 2004 survey of physician executives by the American College of Physician Executives on the topic of disruptive behavior by physicians, 95% of 1,600 respondents reported encountering disruptive behavior on a regular basis. Almost one-third of the respondents reported encountering problems with physician behavior either weekly (14%) or monthly (18%). Furthermore, 83% reported that they had observed disrespect, 51% noted refusals to carry out tasks or duties, 41% had witnessed yelling, 37% reported insults, and 9% noted physical abuse. Seventy percent of respondents indicated that the behavior problems repeatedly involved the same individuals.[6]

Among the limited data available on disruptive behavior among staff positions other than physicians, the Veterans Health Administration (VHA) conducted surveys in 2002 and 2004, and 68% of respondents noted disruptive behavior in nurses.[7] Of course, perceptions of disruptive behavior can also depend on who is observing it. In a VHA survey of operating room (OR) physicians and nurses, 22% of surgeons reported observing disruptive behavior by physicians, while only 12% of anesthesiologists noted it. On the other hand, 21% of OR nurses reported witnessing disruptive physician behavior on a weekly basis.[7]

Who Is Disruptive?

As studies and anecdotal evidence suggest, disruptive behavior is not limited to only one segment of the health care field. Although the literature most frequently discusses disruptive physicians (and research seems to support the notion that the

---

* Most published studies have looked at the hospital setting.

most frequent perpetrators of such behavior are physicians), disruptive behavior is observed between physicians, from physicians toward allied health professionals or nurses, between nurses, from nurses toward technicians or aides, from administrators toward clinical staff, and so on. The potential for disruptive behavior exists in almost all working environments, but the factors that cause an individual to be disruptive are varied and should be taken into consideration by organizations working toward defusing or preventing disruptive behavior in the workplace. Table 1-1, right, lists some of the common behaviors displayed by disruptive staff members.

The Disruptive Physician

The disruptive physician can have the most significant impact on patient care. As defined by the AMA (*see* pages 6–7), disruptive behavior is a "style of interaction with physicians, hospital personnel, patients, family members, or others that interferes with patient care." While there is no one specific profile of a disruptive physician, there are some qualities worth noting.

Joint Commission Resources consultant Thomas Wallace suggests that the high incidence of disruptive behavior among physicians is due in part to the style of education and training they received. For example, during their residencies, many surgeons went through a pyramid program, in which they were placed in an often hostile and highly competitive environment where their very existence in the program was not certain. "These types of programs didn't give surgical residents much time or incentive to work on their teamwork or communication skills," Wallace notes. Although pyramid programs no longer exist, many surgeons and physicians who were trained under them are still in practice, and their perspective and approach still affects the health care work environment.

Also, medical students have been encouraged to think independently, be decisive, and take risks, Wallace adds. While these are important and necessary qualities for a physician to have, it isn't always an easy transition for a new resident who walks into a health care environment that now also demands a team-based approach to care. Wallace notes that there is little training to help new physicians learn the right skills for teamwork. "They are in a competitive, driven environment through years of schooling," Wallace explains. "And then they come to a hospital, where they are now expected to know how to function and communicate well on a team." In his years as a physician executive, Wallace also observed that physicians who exhibit disruptive behavior are often in high-profile positions

---

Table 1-1. Common Behaviors in Disruptive Staff

Inappropriate anger or resentment
- Intimidation
- Abusive language
- Blaming or shaming of others for possible adverse outcomes
- Sarcasm or cynicism
- Threats of violence, retribution, or litigation

Inappropriate words or actions directed toward another person
- Sexual comments or innuendos
- Sexual harassment
- Seductive, aggressive, or assaultive behavior
- Racial, ethnic, or socioeconomic slurs
- Lack of regard for personal comfort or dignity of others

Inappropriate response to patient needs or staff requests
- Late or unsuitable replies to pages or calls
- Unprofessional demeanor or conduct
- Uncooperative, defiant approach to problems
- Rigid, inflexible responses to requests for assistance or cooperation

---

as effective revenue generators for the hospital. "These physicians are often very good at what they do," he notes. This can create a dilemma for health care organizations that rely heavily on their revenue and talent. "The most important factor here is that we don't want the physician to be gone; we want the disruptive behavior to go away," stresses Wallace.

He also notes that all types of licensed independent practitioners—podiatrists, dentists, and so on—should be considered in the same category as physicians when policies and procedures are being developed to deal with disruptive behavior. "This helps create a consistent approach to how independent practitioners are handled with regard to disruptive behavior," Wallace says.

John-Henry Pfifferling, who provides interventional services to physicians who have been reported for disruptive behavior, notes that a disruptive physician often displays behaviors that result in the following negative outcomes:
- Undermining practice morale
- Heightening turnover in the organization
- Stealing from productive activities
- Increasing the risks for ineffective or substandard practice
- Promoting distress among colleagues
- Decreasing synergistic decision making and care
- Ultimately causing harm/distress to the perpetrator and/or his or her family

"The disruptive professional uses his behavior to control or intimidate others," Pfifferling explains.

Unfortunately, some disruptive behavior is the outcome of personality disorders or other undiagnosed conditions. "Anecdotally, I am observing a connection between those physicians I work with who are reported for disruptive behavior and undiagnosed cases of attention deficit/hyperactivity disorder, for example," notes Pfifferling. "For years they have been able to manage their condition and the complexity of their work, but if there is a change in workload or expectation, this can often lead to outbursts and disruptive behavior."

Even more serious than an underlying psychiatric or behavioral disorder is the disruptive behavior that is the outcome of substance abuse. An impaired physician (*see* Sidebar 1-1 on page 6) can cause adverse outcomes in patient care and should be dealt with immediately.

Disruptive physicians, Pfifferling notes, are often narcissistic, perfectionistic, hypercritical, egotistical, manipulative, and usually unaware of their negative impact. "If other staff are intimidated by the physician or afraid of repercussions that could come out of reporting a complaint, their behavior may go unchecked for a long time," Pfifferling says. "I have often met with physicians who had no idea that their behavior was disruptive."

Because of the leadership role that a physician plays on the health care team, his or her disruptive behavior can cause a dangerous domino effect throughout the organization. Grena Porto, R.N., M.S., A.R.M., C.P.H.R.M., senior vice president of Marsh, Inc. (a risk specialist company in Philadelphia), and a member of the Joint Commission's Sentinel Event Advisory Group (which determines the National Patient Safety Goals that are released each year—*see* the Foreword), has seen several incidents of disruptive behavior begetting more disruptive behavior. "It often happens in an OR, where disruptive behavior is on the part of surgeons and physicians that the OR nurses also begin to show disruptive behavior toward each other and the technicians," she explains. "This kind of 'kick the dog' behavior can be detrimental to the proper and safe functioning of an OR and should not be tolerated."

The following two case examples of disruptive behavior are based on real-life incidents:

Fear of Bothering the Physician

Needing to act but not wanting another harassing encounter with the physician, a nurse makes a judgment of the appropriate insulin dose for a patient and administers it. Two hours later, she finds the patient completely unresponsive due to low blood sugar. She administers concentrated injections of glucose and calls for additional emergency help. Despite all attempts to restore the patient to consciousness, he never awakens, and his brain never functions normally again.

Physical Abuse in the OR

During a surgical procedure, the surgeon becomes angry when a particular instrument is not given to him in time. After berating the nurse in front of the rest of the surgical team, he hurls the instrument in her general direction and storms out of the OR. The anesthesiologist follows the surgeon to try to calm him down so the surgery can be concluded. The delay causes a complication for the patient, who dies as a result.

The Disruptive Nurse

Disruptive behavior exhibited by nurses is often different from that of physicians. For example, Porto explains, the climate in some health care organizations among nurses is to "eat their young." "It is not uncommon for some older, very experienced staff nurses to be harsh and pick on the new or inexperienced nurses on their unit," she says. This kind of intimidation can lead to adverse events. Porto illustrates this point with a real-life example:

New on the Night Shift

Two new nurses were working the night shift on a unit with a very experienced but intimidating nurse. The experienced nurse was rude and generally unhelpful to the newer nurses. When a patient who was under the care of the more experienced nurse showed some information in his vital signs that the newer nurses questioned, they chose not to approach the experienced nurse about it for fear of her negative reaction. In the morning, when the physician checked on the patient, it was discovered that the patient had experienced a heart attack. Although the patient was saved, this illustrates how disruptive behavior can impact the ability of staff to provide care.

Also, as previously noted, the recipient of disruptive behavior will sometimes, in turn, show similar behavior toward other staff members. This may include being abusive toward aides, housekeeping staff, or therapists. It can also result in "acting out" beyond the workplace, such as at home or with family members.

The Disruptive Administrator

More subtle and less specific than the disruptive behavior of a physician or nurse, the disruptive behavior of an administrator—or staff member in a leadership role—often involves an unwillingness to champion or support initiatives, regardless of their merit. Other administrators protect certain staff members by refusing to address their reported disruptive behavior. This sends a mixed message—that leadership has a code of conduct for the organization but that some staff members are exempt. Disruptive behavior by administrators can have a detrimental impact on staff morale and could lead to financial costs in the form of staff turnover or missed work days. The following example illustrates one of the ways in which an administrator can be disruptive:

Ignoring the Problem

When a nurse manager brought a concern to the chief medical officer (CMO) about a physician who had been exhibiting a pattern of disruptive behavior toward the nurses on her unit, the CMO listened to the nurse manager's concern but did nothing about the situation. "You know how Bob is," he explained to the manager in a patronizing tone. "We all know he's inappropriate, but he's great friends with the chair of our board, and he's been practicing in the community for 35 years. He's a good doctor, and the patients love him. What am I supposed to do? He'll retire in a few years anyway. Just tell your nurses not to take it personally; in the old days, you guys would just let it roll off your back."

The nurse manager was frustrated by the lack of support and took the issue to the chief nursing officer, but again the problem was unresolved. Everyone stressed that they understood the problem but believed that the physician was protected, untouchable, and too valuable to lose just to "placate" some unhappy staff members. In the meantime, the nurse manager was dealing with an increased incidence of absenteeism, anxiety, and stress among her staff.

While not directly the cause of disruptive behavior, this kind of administrator becomes disruptive when his or her action or inaction does nothing to improve the situation or modify the inappropriate behavior. By refusing (or claiming to be unable) to act, the administrator is not only giving the disruptive staff member the unspoken message that his or her behavior is tolerable and acceptable but causes other staff members to feel more demoralized and certain that their concerns and struggles are considered irrelevant to an uncaring and unsupportive leadership.

Identifying Disruptive Behavior: A Checklist

Organizations can use the checklist on page 12 to identify incidents and the patterns of disruptive behavior. To help identify these trends, review available data from complaint reports, patient satisfaction surveys, medical staff documentation, human resources material, and any other data that may contain information relating to reports of or information about disruptive behavior. Use the checklist to document the number of times reports have been made and the kinds of reports that have been submitted. This will help leaders focus on areas that may require more training and can help staff identify disruptive behavior.

Why Is Managing Disruptive Behavior Necessary and Important?

In 2003–2004, the ISMP surveyed health care workers about workplace intimidation. This study sheds some light on the links between disruptive behavior and safety risks. It found, as stated earlier, that the vast majority of respondents had experienced disruptive behavior in the workplace (88%). In addition, the study noted that 49% of respondents' experiences with intimidation had altered how they handled questions or clarifications about an order. Further, 49% of respondents had felt pressure during the previous year to accept an order, dispense a product, or administer a medication, despite their concerns. In addition, 7% of respondents noted that, in the previous year, a staff member had been involved in a medication error in which intimidation played a role.[8] These numbers show how dangerous disruptive behavior can be and provide further evidence that organizations must tackle the problem.

For Your Consideration

Examples of Disruptive Behavior	Observed, Reputed, Validated, or Documented Cases
• Profane or disrespectful language	
• Demeaning behavior, such as name-calling	
• Sexual comments or innuendo	
• Inappropriate touching, sexual or otherwise	
• Racial or ethnic jokes	
• Outbursts of anger	
• Throwing of instruments, charts, or other objects	
• Criticism of other caregivers in front of patients or other staff	
• Comments that undermine a caregiver's self-confidence in caring for patients	
• Failure to adequately address safety concerns or patient care needs expressed by another caregiver	
• Intimidating behavior that has the effect of suppressing input by other members of the health care team	
• Retaliation against any member of the health care team who has reported an instance of violation of the organization's established code of conduct or who has participated in the investigation of such an incident, regardless of the perceived veracity of the report	

In fact, The Joint Commission, as it developed language on new compliance requirements relating to disruptive behavior, states:

> Safety and quality thrive in an environment that supports working in teams and respecting other people, regardless of their position in the organization. Undesirable behaviors that intimidate staff, decrease morale, or increase staff turnover can threaten the safety and quality of care. These behaviors may be verbal or nonverbal and may involve the use of rude language, threatening manners, or even physical abuse. Anyone who works in the organization can display these disruptive behaviors, including management, clinical and administrative staff, volunteers, licensed independent practitioners, and governing body members. Leaders must be prepared to address such disruptive behavior at any level.

In addition to the demonstrated links between disruptive behavior and patient safety risks, curtailing this type of behavior is important for the sake of civility. In a civil, healthy, supportive work environment, staff are far more willing to work together effectively and to embrace positive change. An individual—or a group of individuals—being allowed to perpetuate abusive behavior can have a demoralizing impact on staff and impair the organization's ability to institute changes, particularly in relation to establishing a culture of safety. Subsequent chapters in this book address the impact of disruptive behavior and lay out steps to establish an effective process to address, prevent, and defuse disruptive behavior.

As the connection between patient safety and disruptive behavior is becoming more clear, this issue is gaining significant attention. One outcome of this realization is that the Joint Commission has released elements of performance (EPs) under Standard LD.3.10 that require an organization to provide an appropriate code of conduct for all members of its staff. The Joint Commission outlines the following EPs from LD.3.10 that must be met for an organization to be in compliance:

4. The [organization] has a code of conduct that defines acceptable and disruptive and inappropriate (**BHC: staff**) behaviors.
5. Leaders create and implement a process for managing disruptive and inappropriate (**BHC: staff**) behaviors.*

Joint Commission Call to Set Expectations for Disruptive Behavior

Table 1-2 on page 14, contains, in its entirety, the forthcoming Joint Commission standard related to establishing a culture of safety. The standard is applicable to the ambulatory care, behavioral health care, critical access hospital, home care, hospital, laboratory, long term care, and office-based surgery programs. Health care organizations are expected to comply with this standard beginning in 2009.

Clearly, an imperative exists to address the issue of disruptive behavior in health care organizations. While the type of behavior differs in different types of organizations, the detrimental impact it can have on staff, the organization, and patient safety is shared. Subsequent chapters in this book address the impact and causes of disruptive behavior, explore ways to effectively defuse disruptive behavior, share examples of how organizations can set up processes and policies to address disruptive behavior, and look at techniques such as conflict resolution to help staff deal with the incidence of disruptive behavior when it crosses their path.

For Your Consideration

1. What steps has your organization taken to establish a culture of safety? What stumbling blocks have you encountered along the way?
2. What steps is your organization taking to educate leaders and staff about disruptive behavior and assess your organization's culture? Who should be involved in this education?

---

* BHC, behavioral health care.

Table 1-2. The Joint Commission's New Disruptive Behavior Elements of Performance Under Standard LD.3.10*

Standard LD.3.10
Leaders create and maintain a culture of safety and quality throughout the organization.

Rationale for LD.3.10
A culture of safety and quality exists when all who work in the organization are focused on excellent performance. Leaders demonstrate their commitment to quality and set expectations for those who work in the organization. Leaders create structures, processes, and programs that allow a culture of safety and quality to flourish. **(AHC, BHC, LAB, LTC, OBS, OME)** Culture can be evaluated in many ways, such as through formal surveys, focus groups, staff interviews, and data analysis.

Safety and quality thrive in a work environment that supports teamwork and respect for other people, regardless of their position in the organization. Disruptive behavior that intimidates staff and affects morale or staff turnover can also harm care. Leaders must address disruptive behavior of individuals working at all levels of the organization, including management, clinical and administrative staff, licensed independent practitioners, and governing body members.

Elements of Performance for LD.3.10
1. Leaders regularly evaluate the culture of safety and quality **(CAH, HAP:** using valid and reliable tools).
2. Leaders prioritize and implement changes identified by the evaluation.
3. All individuals who work in the organization have the opportunity to participate in safety and quality initiatives.
4. The [organization] has a code of conduct that defines acceptable and disruptive and inappropriate **(BHC:** staff) behaviors.
5. Leaders create and implement a process for managing disruptive and inappropriate **(BHC:** staff) behaviors.
6. Leaders provide education that focuses on safety and quality for all individuals.
7. Leaders establish a team approach among all levels of staff.
8. All who work in the organization openly discuss issues of safety and quality.
9. Literature and advisories relevant to patient safety are available to individuals who work in the organization.
10. Leaders define how members of the population served can help manage issues of safety and quality within the organization.

* **AHC,** ambulatory care; **BHC,** behavioral health care; **CAH,** critical access hospital; **HAP,** hospital; **LAB,** laboratory; **LTC,** long term care; **OBS,** office-based surgery; **OME,** home care.

References

1. Pfifferling, J.-H.: Managing the unmanageable: The disruptive physician. *Fam Pract Manag* 4(10):76–8, 83, 87–92, 1997.
2. Porto G., Lauve R.: Disruptive clinician behavior: A persistent threat to patient safety. *Patient Saf QualHealthc* 3(4):16–24, 2006.
3. American Medical Association: *Physicians and Disruptive Behavior.* http://www.ama-assn.org/ama1/pub/upload/mm/21/ disruptive_physician.doc (accessed Apr. 13, 2007).
4. Leape L., Fromson J.: Problem doctors: Is there a system-level solution? *Ann Intern Med* 144(2):107–115, 2006.
5. Institute for Safe Medication Practices: Intimidation: Practitioners speak up about this unresolved problem (Part I). *ISMP Medication Safety Alert* Mar. 11, 2004.
6. Weber D.O.: Poll results: Doctors' disruptive behavior disturbs physician leaders. *Physician Exec* 30(4):6–14, 2004.
7. ECRI: Disruptive practitioner behavior. *HRC* Suppl. A, May 2006.
8. Civility in the health care workplace: Strategies for eliminating disruptive behavior. *Joint Commission Perspectives on Patient Safety* 6(1):1–8, 2006.

For Your Consideration

This work sheet should give an organization a clear picture of its current practices for managing disruptive behavior. Having a clear idea of what processes are already in place will help leaders determine what additional steps, if any, need to be taken. It also provides a helpful snapshot to determine what an organization needs to do to support the establishment of a climate of zero tolerance for disruptive behavior.

Consider: Is your organization promoting a culture of safety? Is your organization tolerant of disruptive behavior? Use the questions below to ascertain the culture of your organization and take stock of your work to date.

Culture of Safety and Patient Safety	
Question	**Response**
1. What patient safety initiatives and measures does your organization have in place? What is your patient safety structure? Do you have a committee? dedicated staff? How long has this structure been in place?	
2. How would you describe your organization's culture? How effectively has it embraced the culture of safety? What measures have you put in place to help establish this culture?	
3. What success stories can you relate about the implementation of a culture of safety? What stumbling blocks are preventing some steps? What revisions or changes to the process should be implemented?	
4. How effectively have you involved staff at all levels and from all disciplines in the safety work? What examples can you share to document this success?	
Disruptive Behavior Process	
Question	**Response**
5. What is your organization's experience with disruptive behavior? Where have incidences of disruptive behavior occurred most often? What seem to be the stressors and triggers that have led to disruptive behavior? What impact has disruptive behavior had on your organization over the past 5 to 10 years?	
6. What is your organization's disruptive behavior management process? If your organization has a medical staff, how does the process for medical staff members and other licensed independent practitioners differ from the process for other staff? How long has it been in place? How effective has it been in managing and defusing disruptive behavior?	
7. Do you have a code of professional conduct? What is the content of the code? Does it clearly distinguish between acceptable and unacceptable behavior? How familiar are staff with the code? How are they oriented to it? Is there any regular training or information shared on the code? Is the information posted anywhere?	
8. What is your process to educate and train staff on disruptive behavior? How familiar are staff with your process? Do staff feel comfortable and empowered to bring concerns and questions to leadership?	

Chapter 2

The Causes and Impact of Disruptive Behavior

In this chapter: Studies have shown that the negative and potentially dangerous effects of disruptive behavior in the health care work environment include lower staff morale, higher turnover rates, and adverse outcomes for patients. This chapter focuses on situations and actions that can lead to disruptive behavior, as well as the impact it can have on patient safety, communication, clinical outcomes, and mortality.

As discussed in Chapter 1, disruptive behavior in the workplace can and does happen, and while it is unacceptable in any environment, its impact on health care can be particularly dire. Disruptive behavior can negatively affect a health care organization in the following ways (among many others): a negative impact on patient safety, which could result in adverse events and unanticipated (and unwelcome) outcomes; diminished staff morale, resulting in staff turnover, fear and resentment, distrust, and human burnout (emotional exhaustion); loss of revenue due to staff turnover or adverse events; and dysfunctional or nonfunctional teamwork or collaboration, which runs contrary to establishing a culture of safety. Disruptive behavior negatively affects a supportive, inclusive, patient safety–oriented workplace and hinders the establishment of a culture of safety. For these important reasons, health care organizations are called to pay close attention to the incidence of disruptive behavior among staff and put in place processes to help prevent or reduce its prevalence.

Disruptive behavior and its impact are not isolated to only one type of health care worker, either. It happens at all levels and is perpetrated and enabled by all types of staff. The causes and triggers of disruptive behavior are varied as well, caused by such things as personality disorders, dysfunctional work environments or teams, stress and anxiety, and substance abuse.

As previously explored, studies suggest that while certain kinds of staff may be more likely than others to perpetrate this behavior, disruptive behavior itself erupts in all staff and displays itself in many forms and ways. Understanding, or at least being aware of, what can cause disruptive behavior and how it affects an organization can help leadership implement proactive measures to help prevent disruptive behavior from happening at all—or at least reduce its occurrence. This chapter explores both of these issues—the causes and impact of disruptive behavior—to help leaders understand why disruptive behavior takes place and why its impact can be so detrimental to the health care environment.

Triggers and Causes of Disruptive Behavior

Almost everyone can relate to having a bad day at work. The reasons, or triggers, for a bad day vary widely and can arise both from within the work environment and from outside pressures—and a really bad day is often the result of several factors in combination. Examples include errors or mistakes committed on the job, conflicts with coworkers, job stress, dissatisfaction with work, lack of sleep, illness, family issues, relationship difficulties, personal problems, and financial troubles. In most cases, having an occasional bad day at work is simply an experience that one learns to live with; however, sometimes stress and a combination of triggers can result in an outburst of disruptive behavior. In health care organizations, disruptive behavior can negatively affect the delivery of safe, high-quality patient care.

For the most part, those having a bad day at work may "act out" to some extent, but they will typically keep their behavior in check or ensure that it does not cause too negative an impact on coworkers. Also, in many cases, when a person acts out disruptively in an isolated manner, he or she typically realizes the inappropriate action immediately and takes steps to improve his or her behavior. An individual's behavior truly becomes disruptive when he or she reacts in such a manner that those working around him or her are unable to perform.

The health care work environment is complex and stressful, and staff members are strongly committed to the mission of improving the health and well-being of the populations they serve. Mistakes or failures in health care can have devastating effects for patients. So it is not surprising that in such a stressful work environment, with such highly driven workers, favorable conditions for episodes and patterns of disruptive behavior exist. A key part of this is that it is generally not a one-time or very rare incident. It is repetitive or cyclical. The cycles can be over months. It is this habitual pattern that moves the behavior into a serious and disruptive pattern that is destructive.

Causes of Disruptive Behavior

Exactly what triggers a particular episode of disruptive behavior is not always clear, but the stress of the clinical environment is often a contributing factor. Another factor could be staffing shortages (particularly in nursing), which have led many organizations to use short-term staffing solutions, including agency or per diem nurses. This approach can actually impair the cohesiveness of a team environment and trigger problems due to culture differences and inadequate staff training.[1] Other possible factors contributing to disruptive behavior include government and regulatory oversight, financial pressures, and increasing liability risks. There are as many causes of disruptive behavior as these are people who perpetrate it, but there are certain common triggers that can cause the behavior, including, but not limited to, the following:

- Unchecked incivility
- Alcohol or substance abuse
- Personality disorders
- Physical, social, or emotional illness
- Overwork and stress
- Personal and/or family strife
- Death of a loved one
- Fear of failure or of making a mistake (particularly in light of the adverse impact that medical errors can have)
- Staffing shortages or staff turnover
- Changes and increasing demands in the health care industry
- An actual or perceived dysfunctional working environment
- Poor, inadequate, or no communication skills
- Self-imposed, peer-imposed, or externally imposed high standards or perfectionistic tendencies ("type A" personality)
- Different perceptions of colleagues' competency based on skills, education, or knowledge

- Cultural differences
- Different educational backgrounds
- Differing work styles
- Poor teamwork skills
- Disruptive behavior itself

For some staff, a combination of such triggers builds up over time, and lead to in disruptive behavior. For others, a single trigger can lead to an almost immediate outburst of unacceptable behavior directed toward those around them. Still other health care workers might not have learned effective ways to communicate their message and, rather than use appropriate channels to express concerns or frustrations, they erupt and vent their frustration on coworkers. The inability to handle conflict and crucial conversations is critical to this because without these tools, staff are more likely to feel unable to cope with disruptive behavior and may further enable it. Staff with these tools are better able to deal with the behavior and confront it.

Incidents of disruptive behavior can also be connected to the traditional structure of health care organizations—particularly hospitals. Historically, a rigid hierarchy existed in which certain positions were invested with vast authority, power, and status, while others had little or no authority but bore great responsibility to carry out the instructions and orders of those in power. An example of this hierarchical structure is the classic physician–nurse relationship. The physician dictated orders, and the nurse was expected to obediently carry them out. Questioning an order was inappropriate and could be met with expressions of annoyance, anger, or derision. Some physicians would simply ignore the question. With an administration that seemed to value the physician more than the nurse, the only way most nurses could function in such an environment was to adapt. Rather than question an order, a nurse might frame a suggestion in a way that made it seem as if it were the physician's idea. This kind of environment tolerated disruptive behavior if it seemed an effective means of getting the job done. The culture of the organization would adapt to the disruptive behavior, and leaders would tell victims that they, too, must accept and adapt to the perpetrator's conduct. Because there were no consequence for the disruptive staff member and no attempts to change his or her behavior, there was no point in trying to address the issue—it was a sink-or-swim mentality.

Rick Croteau, M.D., former executive director for Strategic Initiatives at The Joint Commission, points to strictly hierarchical structures as being perfect breeding grounds for disruptive behavior. "When an organization is essentially hierarchical in nature, it can send a clear message to those at the top of the structure that they are not accountable to those staff who fall underneath them in the hierarchy," he explains. A hierarchical structure is not accommodating to the team-based approach, which often fosters collegial working relationships among staff and promotes collaboration and direct and open two-way communication.

Disruptive behavior can also be self-perpetuating. Beginning a domino effect of undesirable behavior, one staff member on the receiving end of verbal or nonverbal abuse (but with no recourse or means by which to address it) might end up exhibiting disruptive behavior toward others. When an organization refuses to address disruptive behavior, ignores the issue, or instructs staff to "deal with it," this usually causes a toxic work environment and could communicate the message that disruptive behavior in the workplace is supported at the expense of civility.

Another potential cause of disruptive behavior is differing perceptions of the roles and responsibilities of various staff positions and how they should interact. In a recent study of physicians and nurses in the hospital setting, a significant number of physicians seemed to interpret *cooperation* as their being "assisted" by other staff, while nurses viewed cooperation as a more interactive concept.[2] When staff see their roles and responsibilities differently, misunderstandings are likely, which could lead to tension and disruptive behavior.

Teamwork is also perceived differently by various staff members. In a study of health care workers in operating rooms (ORs), the majority of surgical residents (73%) and attending surgeons (64%) reported high levels of teamwork, but only 39% of attending anesthesiologists, 28% of surgical nurses, 25% of anesthesia nurses, and 10% of anesthesia residents reported the same. This study also looked at whether staff valued steep hierarchies (in which junior team members should not question the decisions of senior team members) over a team-based approach, and although 55% of attending surgeons rejected steep hierarchies, a significant number of attending surgeons still perceived a hierarchical structure to be a more effective means of functioning in the OR.[3]

Another cause of disruptive behavior is the changing climate of health care itself. The patient safety movement is encouraging a more team-based approach, improved collaboration, and more skilled communication among staff members. What was once a predominantly hierarchical structure with certain positions in health care given greater importance over others is now evolving into a team-based work environment in which roles and responsibilities are flattening out to accommodate and respect a wider variety of inputs into patient care. But many staff members are still operating between these styles of working; they were trained under the more hierarchical approach and yet are asked to now foster a team-based approach. Not everyone is happy with the change or in agreement with it. This situation can send mixed messages and leave some individuals in a difficult position due to poor communication skills or a lack of training in teamwork. It could also lead to tension over different philosophies concerning what is and is not appropriate or necessary in a health care environment. One major cause is the legal system that holds the hospital or the physician responsible, leading to physicians sometimes feeling that if things are not done as they direct, they are responsible and reported to the National Practitioner Data Bank. This pressure and being held liable by our legal system helps perpetuate this hierarchy.

These changes reflect the evolving climate in health care, and organizations are scrambling to provide effective education and training to help their staff make the transition to a culture of safety. Still, some clinicians, though absolutely committed to providing safe, high-quality care, feel overwhelmed by the rapidly changing status quo and may sometimes overreact when they perceive that they are losing control over their own work and work style.

Examples of Triggers

Although there is no justification for disruptive behavior in the health care workplace, it is important to understand why such behavior occurs and what triggers it. This section presents four scenarios that provide ideas on the origins of some disruptive behavior. Questions for discussion and consideration follow each scenario.

Sowing the Seeds of Disruptive Behavior:
From Medical Student to New Physician

This scenario follows the education and training of a new physician and portrays the mixed messages, inadequate (or nonexistent) training on teamwork and communication, and other elements that can trigger disruptive behavior by a physician.

A new medical student begins his first day at a renowned medical school. Many years of effort have lead up to this day. The student is confident, driven, competitive, and intelligent. His is a technical mind with a strong affinity for science, and all indications are that he will make a competent, capable physician.

The student is fully aware that he faces at least another eight years of training and residency, but he is confident that he possesses the discipline, intelligence, and commitment to succeed. He also knows that should he successfully navigate the series of challenges before him, a secure, well-paying career as a physician awaits him. Along with that career will come such privileges as respect, leadership, and opportunity.

His ultimate goal of becoming a physician has been at the forefront of his plans for years. Competitive by nature, he enjoys excelling at any challenge placed before him. During his years of education up to this point, he had a reasonable rapport with his fellow students, but he always viewed them as competition and as a result kept them at a distance.

The student's career path is laid out before him, but the years to come are filled with hard work. Rigorous coursework, examinations, a competitive environment, and long hours are the norm. He also receives a cultural education—that of the medical culture. Both directly and indirectly, the medical student is trained to be independent, confident, decisive, and scientifically grounded. Inherent in this educational process—and thus firmly ingrained on the psyche of this focused medical student—is the high value placed on the ability to make accurate diagnoses based on the knowledge, experience, and information gleaned from schooling and residency. A competent physician should be able to treat his or her patients without needing to constantly refer to other staff for instruction or guidance, he learns. A physician needs to function as a self-sufficient source of information and clinical decision-making know-how; the climate, pace, and atmosphere of modern Western medicine demands this.

During residency, the young physician learns by example. He observes several of his mentoring physicians employ a derogatory, abrasive, and abrupt tone with those around them—particularly toward nurses and junior physicians. Although he is surprised by this behavior at first, he notes that no one seems to penalize these physicians. In fact, everyone else seems to adapt to their particular work style.

As he moves into his new role as a full-fledged physician, he notes the changing expectations placed upon him. As a physician, he is not only expected to make effective clinical decisions about patient care, he is now also expected to do so in conjunction with a number of other staff members. He knows that, although the physician drives the clinical care decisions, the care provided to the patient is not carried out by the physician alone. But his experience, education, and training have given him the impression that he is at the top of the tree, and all decisions are his to make. The other members of the "team" serve only to carry out his orders.

This newly minted physician now finds that he often has to work with a team to get the job done. Medical school taught him to be independent, and yet the health care environment requires considerable interdependence. This proves challenging at times because so much of what he has achieved so far has been through his own hard work. Now some degree of his success as a physician will depend on how well those around him do their jobs.

Up to now, he has received mixed messages about how teamwork in the health care environment should function. With no real training in this area during medical school, he picked up most of what he knows about teamwork during residency. Some of his mentoring physicians reminded him that he was the "captain of the charge," his orders and decisions were paramount, and the "support staff" around him simply served to carry out those orders and do them skillfully. Other mentoring physicians reminded him that it was always in his best interest to be "good" to his nurses and not take them for granted. Above all, he learned much by observing how his mentoring physicians interacted with other staff.

He also observed a pattern of behavior that seemed connected to physician skill. Often, the best clinicians, those who were most respected by their peers and other staff for their outstanding skills as physicians, did not possess the interpersonal skills necessary for working well with other staff members. Yet, he noted, the nurses and other staff around those physicians interacted differently with them than they did with other physicians.

The health care organizations with which the physician is now affiliated value his work but also have expectations for him. These expectations appear in different ways. When he is granted admitting privileges at a hospital, he is expected to adhere to the bylaws established by the medical staff of that institution. When he becomes a full-time staff member of that institution, he is also expected to follow the guidelines of the human resources department and adhere to a code of conduct that requires a kind of Golden Rule for all staff—that they treat each other with respect and professionalism.

The medical student—now a physician—is expected to do two things at the same time: be a confident, well-educated clinician who can think on his own feet with effective decision-making skills and work well within a team-oriented framework in an ethical and appropriate manner. This seems logical to the new physician, but at times, balancing these two is not straightforward.

Some days prove challenging for the physician. In his well-ordered mind, the practice of medicine should follow a consistent path, but in the day-to-day reality of a living, breathing health care organization, the actual practice sometimes deviates from those expectations. Also, he carries the assumption that the staff around him approach their work in the same way he does, and he finds himself befuddled by the varying approaches (and priorities) that other staff members have toward the work.

After a number of years on the job, the physician becomes more frustrated and annoyed by what he sees as inadequacies in the staff around him, the shifting priorities and demands of a seemingly ineffective leadership, and an increasing demand to generate more revenue. His competitive nature and heightened fear of failure also contribute to his growing frustration with the work environment. Further, due to his demanding work schedule (and his own inability to slow down), his family life is in turmoil.

Coupled with all these changes in the physician's perception and personal life is a growing change in mood and temperament. The staff who work with him have always been aware of his "type A" personality and his work style, but they now note a growing trend of rudeness, impatience, and occasional outbursts. Newer nurses are intimidated by him, and everyone seems to steel themselves against his criticisms, which are growing increasingly uncivil. After repeated incidents over the course of six months, including several officially filed complaints and the concern expressed by a patient's family who witnessed the physician berating a nurse, the chief medical officer meets with him to discuss his behavior.

This new physician began his career with high expectations for success while recognizing that there would be challenges along the way. How he responded to those challenges throughout his career was influenced by his personality, his work style and communication ability, and his approach to teamwork and the work environment

The new physician in this first scenario is driven, capable, and dedicated. His training and commitment lead him to become a fine physician, but he finds that he needs more than that to be effective in the health care work environment. That environment requires additional skills (effective teamwork and communication, for example) to help him understand and deal with the interpersonal dynamics of working in a team-oriented atmosphere. If he can acquire such skills and adapt to this new work style, he can help ensure a smooth, supportive, and nondisruptive working environment. But because he has difficulty adapting to this environment, the physician's behavior becomes more disruptive over time. Trigger points include the behavior of his mentors, from whom he learns that behavior now considered disruptive was actually an effective way to get the job done; and his lack of training in effective communication and teamwork, which make it difficult for him to appreciate those who work around him or to help him use effective means to produce results.

For Your Consideration

1. In this example, the medical student is faced with mixed messages about how he should behave as a physician in a hospital. What examples of mixed messages have you observed being absorbed by your new staff in the organization? Brainstorm ways to eliminate, remedy, or clarify these mixed messages.

2. What additional triggers or causes could have affected this medical student as he navigated residency? What elements stand out for you as possible causes of disruptive behavior at a later date?

3. If you were intervening with a staff member who was behaving in this manner, what would you do? List some steps that you would take to intervene.

In his work with disruptive physicians, John-Henry Pfifferling, Ph.D., director of the Center for Professional Well-Being, based in North Carolina, has noted a number of common triggers that could cause disruptive behavior by physicians in specific specialties. In the following two scenarios, he shares examples of triggers for the general surgical specialty and examples of triggers for an oncologist.

Scheduling and Staffing Issues for the Surgeon

Jane Smith is an experienced and capable general surgeon who is known for her abrasive manner and abrupt tone, particularly when faced with an unusual or atypical case. One week, while on call, a particularly tough case comes up that Dr. Smith knows will take a long time and involve a number of potential issues that could result in postoperative complications. It isn't that Dr. Smith is incapable of performing the surgery, but she worries that the infrequency of having to perform this particular surgery might result in her needing extra help or cause her to make a mistake.

Dr. Smith has performed surgeries at General Hospital for a number of years and has come to know the OR staff well. She knows that a procedure as complicated as this one requires that she feel comfortable and well supported in the OR. She makes a point to stress with the scheduling staff at the hospital that she wants specific staff members scheduled with her. The schedulers take the message and note that they will do what they can to accommodate the request.

On the morning of the surgery Dr. Smith enters the hospital and begins her prep work in the OR. She immediately notices that the staff scheduled are not who she requested. To make matters worse, they are new staff and relatively unseasoned in the OR. Dr. Smith takes this information negatively and walks briskly to address the issue with the OR coordinator. She addresses the coordinator in a loud voice, stating that she had specifically requested an experienced person. The coordinator begins to speak in response to Dr. Smith's concerns, but she is cut off. Dr. Smith shakes her head, throws the chart down on the coordinator's desk in an abrupt manner, mutters an insulting comment under her breath (though loud enough for the coordinator and those around her to hear) about the "idiots" that she has to deal with, and storms back to the OR.

The newer staff are greeted in the OR with a volatile reception. Dr. Smith has regained some control, but she is clearly still aggravated. The surgeon remarks on every action the staff take in a sarcastic and disparaging manner. While most of the staff are new, the anesthesiologist is experienced and has observed this behavior in Dr. Smith on a few occasions. Not eager to confront her mood, he focuses on his task and offers reassuring glances to the new staff who look nervous and intimidated.

The surgery is performed adequately, but there are problems. Dr. Smith berates the staff for everything from handing her the wrong instruments at the wrong time to not moving fast enough. Throughout the surgery, she offers disparaging comments about the "incompetence" of those around her.

When the surgery is over and it appears to have been successful, Dr. Smith seems calmer but still shows signs of stress. She leaves the OR without a word. Within a few minutes of her departure, one of the nurses—a particularly young one—bursts into tears while she discusses the experience with another nurse, trying to understand what she "did wrong." Over the next few weeks, the nurse calls in sick repeatedly and is observably anxious and uncomfortable at work when she does come in. When she is scheduled for another surgery with the same surgeon, she goes to her manager to request a reassignment.

A Day of Bad News in Oncology

Dr. Bill Jones is an experienced oncologist who runs a successful oncology clinic. Dr. Jones has maintained a busy schedule for years, and the patients and families who receive his care appreciate his calm, knowledgeable demeanor. Recently Dr. Jones and his wife learned that she has breast cancer.

Dr. Jones could be best described as unemotional and stoic. He is rarely found socializing with the staff in his practice, typically talking only when it involves giving an order. As a result, only one or two of his colleague physicians actually knows about his wife's illness.

One particularly busy day in the practice, Dr. Jones has had the duty of seeing patients to deliver bad news about their health. The weight of this is not lost on Dr. Jones, particularly as he is navigating his own personal struggle. After these visits, he goes to sit in his office for a while before continuing to see patients.

He is interrupted by a knock on the door, and one of the nurses pops her head in to ask a question. From his perspective, this question seems unnecessary, particularly considering the weight of his day. Dr. Jones mutters a response, and the nurse leaves the room. Dr. Jones then heads to his first appointment, and before he can get to the first patient, an assistant stops him and tells him that a local pharmacist is on the phone, with a question about a prescription. Dr. Jones stops walking, inhales sharply through his nose, and tells the assistant to "deal" with it.

He enters the room of the next patient. He tries to answer the patient's questions but is distracted. After a few minutes, he walks from the room and back to his office. Not a minute after sitting down, there is a knock on the door. He says "Come in" in a sharp voice, and it is the same assistant who had been on the phone with the local pharmacy to clarify a medication order. The pharmacy has called back again.

"Didn't I tell you to deal with it?" Dr. Jones asks the assistant. "I don't have the time to deal with this sort of nonsense. While Dr. Jones does not raise his voice, his body language is tight, and his hands are clenched as he looks at the assistant. The assistant backs out of the office and closes the door.

Not knowing what else to do and afraid to talk to anyone else, the assistant goes back to the phone and confirms with the pharmacy that the order (which seems like far too high of a dose to the pharmacist) is correct and that the doctor confirmed it.

That night, the physician is phoned by one of his colleagues, who informs him that the patient for whom he wrote the prescription in question had an adverse medication reaction that forced him to go to the emergency room for treatment. While the patient is going to make a full recovery, the error could have resulted in something much worse.

For Your Consideration

1. In these two scenarios, a number of factors contributed to the disruptive behavior, and the individuals involved were "set off" by different triggers and stressors. What stressors in your organization could potentially lead to disruptive behavior?
2. Did the caregivers in these two scenarios have any other options for responding to the disruptive behavior? What processes does your organization have in place to address this kind of behavior?

These two scenarios illustrate an important point that organization leaders must consider when developing policies and procedures for addressing disruptive behavior: Many different events and situations can serve as triggers for disruptive behavior, and something that might be ignored or considered trivial by one person could lead another to inappropriate conduct. Moreover, the same or similar events that a health care worker has dealt with appropriately in the past might cause him or her to behave disruptively under more stressful conditions.

For Your Consideration

Consider the different areas of care, treatment, and services that your organization provides (for example, a home care organization that provides home health, hospice, and respiratory care services). Then consider the kinds of triggers or outbursts of disruptive behavior that take place in those areas. How do they differ? How have staff handled the disruptive behavior in different situations?

A Pattern of Horizontal Disruptive Behavior:

Nurse–Nurse

Mary Johnson is an experienced night shift nurse who has worked in the field for 15 years. She is the most senior nurse on the shift, and her experience and skills make her a valuable resource to the hospital and unit. She has endured years of disruptive behavior from physicians and changing management styles in administration. She has attended the required training courses on the performance improvement flavor of the month. She has seen her paperwork and recording workload increase. She has lived with the difficulties that staff shortages have brought and has kept abreast of the many changes in regulations and policies she has seen in her years as a nurse. Her load of patients has increased, too, yet she has endured.

Her hope of being promoted to nurse manager has not materialized, however, and this perplexes Mary. She believes that she is competent and capable, but she perceives that management prefers the "smooth talkers" on staff, who seem to be moving ahead of her. The latest blow is when Julie, a younger nurse with fewer years on the job, is promoted to a vacant nurse manager position. Mary is told that this promotion has no bearing on her performance but is the result of Julie's qualifications and training. Even so, Mary takes this personally.

When Julie starts in her new position, Mary resists her directions. She feels that Julie has not earned the position and is not as competent as she is. At meetings, she makes negative comments about almost everything Julie says, and outside meetings, she gossips about Julie and her work style. Every request from Julie makes Mary feel like she is being controlled and "picked on."

During a shift, Julie lets Mary know that the wife of one of her patients is worried that her husband is feeling more pain. Mary has always been strongly committed to her patients, and she goes to help the patient immediately. But while she cares for her patient, she feels a growing sense of frustration.

Her anger continues to grow as she walks back to the nurses' station. Julie is waiting there and asks how the patient is doing. Mary can contain herself no longer. "What, do you think I'm stupid? that I can't handle the situation? If I wasn't in one of your stupid meetings, I would have been able to check on them sooner. Are you trying to do my job for me? Do you think I can't handle it?"

As Mary continues her tirade, she does not realize that a few patients and family members are standing in the hall, watching the outburst. The next day, one of the family members of a patient files a complaint with the hospital, expressing concern over seeing such a display.

For Your Consideration

1. What are some of the stressors that you can identify in this scenario?
2. If a nurse manager in your organization finds himself or herself in a situation such as the one described in this scenario, how is that person mentored and trained to handle it?
3. What could have been done sooner to help address Mary's issues?

Each area of health care can have different triggers and stressors that can trigger disruptive behavior, and these scenarios show just a few. Organizations should examine the scope of care, treatment, and services they provide in order to identify potential triggers. By looking at data collected from reports filed or disciplinary actions taken for disruptive behavior, surveying staff, and considering anecdotal reports, leaders can begin to understand the situation in their organizations and then develop policies to address the behavior. These data will not provide a complete picture of every kind of stressor or trigger within an organization, but proactive measures can be put in place to address other issues that might arise. Table 2-1 on page 26 provides a worksheet to help reflect on the kinds of disruptive behavior that can occur in a specific health care organization. Table 2-2 on page 27 is a worksheet to help map out the kinds of care, treatment, and services offered and the types of stressors or triggers that can cause disruptive behavior.

The Impact of Disruptive Behavior

Disruptive behavior can lower staff morale, increase turnover, damage teamwork, delay an organization's efforts to establish a culture of safety, and lead to adverse events. For example, in a 2004 Institute for Safe Medication Practices (ISMP) study, found that 49% of pharmacists responding reported that their experiences with intimidation as a result of disruptive behavior had caused them to alter the way they handled clarifications or questions about medication orders.[4] This response to disruptive behavior is typical of the negative impact it can have on staff morale and effective teamwork. This section explores the many ways that disruptive behavior can affect staff, health care organizations, and patient safety.

Impact on Staff Morale

One of the most common effects of disruptive behavior is its negative impact on staff morale. In a study of nurses in the United States, Canada, England, Scotland, and Germany, 41% reported that they were dissatisfied with their jobs, and they attributed that dissatisfaction in part to verbal abuse in the workplace.[5] Individuals on the receiving end of disruptive behavior may experience the following personal reactions[6]:

- Stress
- Anxiety
- Emotional withdrawal
- Fear
- Resentment
- Poor communication
- Feelings of worthlessness
- A breakdown in collaborative efforts
- Damaged self-esteem
- Blame shifting
- Reduced initiative

With appropriate and immediate interventions, most staff can recover from an isolated incident of disruptive behavior and its effects. If the situation is left unresolved or is ignored, however, it can have a long-term affect, possibly including the continuation of the behavior by the original perpetrator and the expansion of disruptive conduct by leading the victim to act out as well.

When a staff member is beginning to feel the effects of disruptive behavior, it inevitably begins to affect those around him or her as well. This ends up affecting staff morale in general. Consider the following example:

Sarah has been working as a nursing assistant in a busy ambulatory medical office for six months. She comes to the position with experience and solid skills. Her demeanor is pleasant, and patients feel at ease with her. One of the partners in the practice has been consistently rude and abrupt with her, even berating her on a number of occasions. Sarah mentions the situation to her supervisor, and although the supervisor is sympathetic, she tells Sarah, "That's just how he is; we just work around it." The supervisor also tells her to try to let it "roll off her back." She assures Sarah that she will eventually get used to the way that physician behaved and will learn to anticipate when he is about to have an outburst.

Sarah tries this technique, but every time she sees this physician, she becomes anxious and nervous, worried that anything she might do could cause him to explode at her. After a while, Sarah becomes increasingly uncomfortable in the work environment, and her productivity is impaired. She begins to second-guess everything she does and begins making small mistakes that are noticeable to others.

This scenario illustrates how repeated incidents of unchecked disruptive behavior can affect staff morale. What is also troubling about this example is that other staff who have been affected by the behavior have learned to cope with it and were encouraging coworkers to do the same. By ignoring the issue, those around the victim of disruptive behavior become almost complicit in the behavior and exacerbate the victim's feeling of hopelessness. When staff morale is impaired to such a degree, the environment itself grows increasingly toxic, and the organization find it more difficult to make improvements.

Table 2-1. Anecdotal Experiences with Disruptive Behavior

Using this grid, reflect on and document the kinds of disruptive behaviors you have encountered in health care organizations.

Area/Department Where Events Took Place	Types of Staff Members Involved	Description of Event

Table 2-2. Identifying Stressors or Triggers in a Health Care Organization

Consider the events and situations that you can identify as triggers for disruptive behavior in your organization. Examine any data that have been collected about incidents of disruptive behavior in your organization in the form of filed complaints (and the documented process that followed to investigate the event), anecdotal accounts, direct observation, results from internal surveys, and so on. Examples are provided in the header row.

Stressor/Trigger (overwork/stress)	Description of This Disruptive Behavior (yelling and abuse in the unit)	How Often This Trigger Has Caused Disruptive Behavior (daily, weekly)	Data Source for This Trigger (filed reports, direct observation, etc.)	Department/Staff Involved in This Trigger (ICU, OR, nurses, pharmacists, etc.)

Impact on Staff Turnover

One of the costliest impacts of disruptive behavior is high staff turnover. In the preceding example, after a prolonged experience with demoralizing treatment in the workplace, Sarah would probably leave her position and seek employment elsewhere. In a busy workplace, losing trained, competent staff members further harms staff morale. These are not isolated incidents. In a Veterans Health Administration (VHA) study, about 31% of all respondents noted that they knew of a nurse who had left a hospital as a result of disruptive physician behavior.[7]

Research shows that the cost of replacing staff is in the tens of thousands of dollars, with the total cost based on the type of position.[6] The financial impact of staff turnover extends to many areas, depending on how difficult it is to replace a particular position. Clearly, losing staff members due to disruptive behavior can have a far greater impact than just upsetting one individual. It can disturb the balance needed in an organization to ensure that safe, high-quality care is being delivered.

Impact on Teamwork and Collaboration

Related to staff morale is the impact that disruptive behavior has on teamwork and collaboration. Typically, the perpetrator of disruptive behavior is uncomfortable with the idea of teamwork, or at least he or she often disagrees with the organization's philosophy of teamwork. Because teamwork relies on trust and mutual respect, the disruptive behavior of one or more staff members can severely hamper its success. Partnered with effective teamwork and collaboration is effective communication, which is a cornerstone of preventing sentinel events. The Joint Commission has reported that 24% of sentinel events could be attributed to a problem with nurse staffing, communication gaps, a lack of teamwork, or other "human factors."[8]

The following example illustrates how an organization's cohesiveness and sense of teamwork can disintegrate when a climate of disruptive behavior is tolerated or left unchecked.

A successful oncology clinic in a suburban area of a large city had undergone some recent changes in staffing by adding two new physicians to its group. In addition, to accommodate its growing success and load of patients, the group had recently moved into a larger facility. Before the move, the clinic had operated smoothly, with

the physicians maintaining a collegial attitude with each other and the nursing staff working close together in a spirit of teamwork. There was a sense of fun in the clinic, too, with the staff taking advantage of key holidays and events to celebrate in the office.

However, things began to change with the addition of new medical staff and the move to new facilities. It became clear from the outset that one of the senior physicians in the practice did not get along with one of the newer ones. Not only were their work styles different, but their personalities and personal philosophies varied widely as well. To make things more challenging, there was no clear, solid leadership in the clinic among the physicians. Before the staffing increase, there had been three physicians, and they had been able to work together informally to make decisions, and because their work styles and approaches were similar, they rarely had differences of opinion. But things were different now. In the absence of a solid, effective leader and a clear set of guidelines on how the practice members would interact, these differences had gone unresolved, and the tension kept growing. Both physicians were acting disruptively toward each other, and at times, due to the unresolved differences, began to exhibit disruptive behavior toward the nursing staff as well. Attempts by either side to discuss the differences resulted only in outbursts or cold indifference, and without a neutral facilitator to help smooth the interaction, both physicians felt worse than before the discussion. This situation had not gone unnoticed by staff. Not only did the nurses feel the sting of occasional and unwarranted outbursts directed toward them, but the tension had begun to spill over into how the nurses interacted with each other, with the nurse of one physician seeming to act out with the same negativity toward the other physician's nurse in an attempt to protect or defend that physician.

After a year of unresolved differences and repeated disruptive incidents, the physicians now opted to avoid each other entirely—choosing to use intermediaries to communicate. Rather than use appropriate channels to resolve the issues, the physicians chose to "vent" about each other to selected physician colleagues. At times, even the nurses were drawn into the silent siege by being subject to complaints or negative comments from one physician to the other. The nursing staff had been damaged by this tension as well—and rather than enjoy the close teamwork they had once shared, all staff felt like they were "walking on eggshells" around these physicians. The sense of fun and cooperation in the practice was gone, and some nurses felt ostracized for "protecting their physician."

Impact on Patient Safety

By far the most potentially dangerous impact of disruptive behavior is its effect on patient safety. The numbers speak for themselves in the following excerpts from recent key studies on the impact of disruptive behavior on patient safety:

- Rosenstein and O'Daniel found in a 2005 VHA survey that "disruptive behaviors raised stress and frustration levels, affected levels of concentration, and impeded communication, collaboration, and transfer of information, all of which are crucially important for optimizing outcomes of patient care."[7] They also found that 19% of respondents to their survey noted that they were aware of a specific adverse event that occurred as a result of disruptive behavior, and 78% of those surveyed felt that the adverse event was preventable.[7]

- In the same study, 94% of respondents believed that disruptive behavior could have a negative impact on patient safety, and 46% reported an awareness of a specific event related to disruptive behavior that could have resulted in an adverse event. In addition, respondents noted a link between disruptive behavior and impaired quality (68%), adverse events (67%), medical errors (67%), compromises in safety (58%), and mortality (28%).[7]

- In a 2003 survey, the ISMP found that 75% of responding pharmacists had asked a colleague to help them interpret a prescription rather than approach an intimidating physician for clarification. In addition, and probably most alarmingly, 7% of respondents reported that they had been involved in a medication error during the previous year in which they claimed that intimidation played a role.[4]

In a recently noted National Strategic Partnership Forum listserve discussion thread, patients and family members posted their observations of disruptive behavior by clinicians that had had adverse impacts on the care delivered.[6]

To actually ensure a patient-safe health care organization and one that is truly embracing the concept of a culture of safety,

preventable causes of adverse events must be reduced as much as possible. This includes the impact of disruptive behavior on patient safety. In a patient safety–focused organization, civility, collaboration, skilled communication, effective teamwork, staff retention efforts, staff encouragement, and positive feedback play important roles. In such an environment, there is no room for the toxicity that can come from disruptive behavior.

Impact of Disruptive Behavior on Various Staff

Staff are affected by disruptive behavior in different ways. In his research and work with disruptive behavior, John-Henry Pfifferling outlines in the following ways that staff are affected by disruptive behavior[6]:

Impact of Disruptive Behavior on Staff
- Withholding of information (due to intimidation or fear)
- Staff cover-up of mistakes of higher-level staff for fear of retribution from exposing mistakes
- Reduced initiative
- Reduced morale
- Reduced self-esteem
- Interstaff blaming and dysfunction
- Harassment and lawsuits stemming from anger
- Increased turnover
- Decreased commitment to public relations for the organization

Impact of Disruptive Behavior on Peers or Coworkers
- Chronic fatigue/complaints
- Psychological and illness absenteeism
- Incomplete and dysfunctional communication, leading to inadequate teamwork
- Dumping on staff and patients
- Premature turnover
- Reduced creativity and innovative problem solving
- Heightened risk and litigation as a result of partner liability (for physicians)
- Increased paperwork and "problem colleague" meetings (for physicians)
- Lawsuit fears and anxiety (due to "threats" from a disruptive physician) (for physicians)
- Corrective or cover-up activities
- Sabotage

Impact of Disruptive Behavior on Administration

- Increased risk of staff or employee lawsuits
- Increased time consumed counseling disgruntled staff, peers, and patients/family members
- Wasted time protecting staff from involvement with disruptive physician
- Dramatic increase in administrator turnover (as a result of not dealing with disruptive behavior)
- Increased psychosomatic risk
- Increased time spent putting out fires and reactive public relations
- Increased time spent on staff recruitment and retention due to increased turnover related to disruptive behavior
- Expensive adversarial processes
- Increased time spent on sexual harassment issues
- Conflict management time spent with all affected individuals
- Increased expenses spent on trying to satisfy "demands" of a disruptive individual
- Time, energy, and expenses engaged in the confrontation process
- Time, energy, and expenses spent in the rehabilitation process

In addition to examining the ways that disruptive behavior can affect staff, it is important to consider how disruptive staff members are affected by their own behavior, which Pfifferling outlines in the following list[6]:

- Potential loss of employment or, if applicable, privileges
- Increased risk of lawsuits from disgruntled patients/family
- Isolation from colleagues or coworkers
- Increased workload because colleagues or coworkers will not assist
- Difficulty finding other employment
- Increased legal costs (to defend allegations)
- Heightened personal morbidity risk
- Decreased social network
- Alienation from administration and its support

When confronted with their own disruptive behavior, some individuals react with surprise. Thomas Wallace, M.D., J.D., M.B.A., consultant for Joint Commission Resources, notes: "It's not unusual to interact with a person who has been reported for disruptive behavior—and the reports will often point to more than one instance—and they seem genuinely surprised that their behavior has been viewed as a problem.

This is often due to the fact that the disruptive behavior can be so intimidating to staff, and the fear of reprisal so great, that it can take a long time for the behavior to be reported through formal channels. In the meantime, because the behavior went unchecked, the offended person just assumes it was considered acceptable to the organization. "The reports often come when tolerance for the behavior has reached its limit and enough staff have grown fed up with the behavior," Wallace says. Regardless of the angle from which the issue is considered, disruptive behavior in a health care organization leaves no one untouched. As studies are now making clear, there are direct links between disruptive behavior and negative outcomes in the delivery of care, treatment, and services. The imperative to address disruptive behavior in the health care workplace has never been more pressing.

📝 For Your Consideration

1. Has your organization seen the impact of disruptive behavior? How has it been demonstrated (for example, financial costs, loss of a good staff member)?
2. Have you seen or become aware of any adverse outcomes or near misses ("good catches") that could be linked to disruptive behavior? What happened? What lessons were learned from the experience?
3. When dealing with both a disruptive staff member and an individual (or group of individuals) affected by the behavior, how has the organization dealt with the issue?

References

1. Porto G., Lauve R.: Disruptive clinician behavior: A persistent threat to patient safety. *Patient Saf Qual Healthc* 3(4):16–24, 2006.
2. Skjorshammer M.: Co-operation and conflict in a hospital: Interprofessional differences in perception and management of conflicts. *J Interprof Care* 15:7–18, 2001.
3. Pizzi L., Goldfarb N., Nash D.: *Crew Resource Management and Its Applications in Medicine.* http://www.ahrq.gov/clinic/ptsafety/pdf/chap44.pdf (accessed Apr. 14, 2007).
4. Institute for Safe Medication Practices: Intimidation: Practitioners speak up about this unresolved problem (Part I). *ISMP Medication Safety Alert* Mar. 11, 2004.
5. Aiken L.H., et al.: Nurses' reports on hospital care in five countries. *Health Aff* 20(3):43–53, 2001.

6. Pfifferling J.-H.: The disruptive physician. *Physician Exec* 25(2):56–61,1999.

7. Rosenstein A., O'Daniel M.: Disruptive behavior in the perioperative arena. *J Am Coll Surg* 203(1):96–105, 2006.

8. www.jointcommission.org/sentinelevents/statistics (accessed Aug. 14, 2007).

Chapter 3

Defusing Disruptive Behavior

In this chapter: This chapter discusses ways to defuse disruptive behavior and considers the various roles that staff can and should play in that process. It also provides an overview of Joint Commission standards that offer related and direct guidance on what to do when disruptive behavior takes place, particularly the new elements of performance under Joint Commission Standard LD.3.10, which delineate the need for a process to deal with disruptive behavior. This chapter also includes examples of what other health care organizations have done to manage disruptive behavior.

Previous chapters have explored what disruptive behavior is in the context of the health care environment, considered what causes or triggers disruptive behavior among different staff, and looked at the negative impact disruptive behavior has on the work environment and patient safety. This chapter considers what steps can be taken to defuse disruptive behavior and how to deal with its impact on staff in a positive, effective way. It also provides examples of how health care leaders countrywide have dealt with eruptions of disruptive behavior in their organizations and what steps they have put in place to minimize its reoccurrence. It also includes a helpful chart of Joint Commission standards related to the issue of disruptive behavior from different angles and provides a framework for dealing with this issue.

Cleaning Up the Mess: Life After a Disruptive Episode

It's unlikely that an organization has not had to deal with some type of disruptive behavior and its impact. While there are informal moments when a colleague intervenes with a disruptive clinician and can help defuse the situation, there are also situations in which a staff member files an official complaint with his or her manager about someone's disruptive behavior,

and a more formal process will have to begin. It can be helpful to have a process mapped out or considered before a disruptive behavior incident so that leadership is well prepared to deal with the situation and help defuse it effectively. How that process is laid out, who should be involved, and what steps can and should be taken depend partly on the dynamics of the organization, but some consistent principles should be in place. In addition, steps should be put in place to educate staff on the process so that they are aware of what will take place and how they can be involved.

The Joint Commission Standards and Disruptive Behavior

Chapter 1 introduced the complete standard, rationale, and elements of performance (EPs) for Standard LD.3.10, the newly revised Leadership standard that directly lays out the Joint Commission's expectations for organizations to deal with disruptive behavior. There are additional standards that relate to the issue as well. While not all of these standards apply to all types of health care organizations (for example, MS.4.30 is a hospital and critical access hospital standard only), they provide a helpful framework for consideration when mapping out a comprehensive system to deal with the issue. Chapter 4 explores more fully the establishment and progression of a zero-tolerance policy and work environment as they relate to disruptive behavior, but this chapter helps to set the ground rules for what is and is not considered acceptable and how to handle situations that emerge, both informally and formally.

In the following sections, the various standards and their related EPs are explored from the perspective of disruptive behavior. In addition, Table 3-1, pages 34–36, provides a helpful list of standards and EPs that relate to some degree to disruptive behavior and the processes that need to be in place to help defuse or prevent it.

Table 3-1. Joint Commission Standards and EPs Related to Disruptive Behavior

The following table includes standards and EPs related, to various extents, to the organization's need to manage disruptive behavior. These standards appear in the "Provision of Care, Treatment, and Services" (PC), "Leadership" (LD), "Management of Human Resources" (HR), and "Medical Staff" (MS)* chapters of the accreditation manuals. EPs or bulleted items within an EP have been italicized strictly for editorial reasons to aid the reader in locating the most pertinent points as they relate to the issue of disruptive behavior.

> **Note:** Some of the standards and elements of performance referenced in this table do not apply to all types of health care settings. Organizations should consult the latest updates from their applicable accreditation manuals for the most up-to-date language and information. In addition, while this table highlights particular issues that relate to disruptive behavior, organizations should not assume that the direct issue of disruptive behavior is being scored under more than one standard. *The only standard where this issue is directly referenced and scored is at standard LD.3.10.* The connections made in this table are only for the purpose of this publication as a means to explore the issues that relate to the broader topic of disruptive behavior and should not be construed as compliance requirements for accreditation purposes.

Standard Number	Language of the Standard	Related Elements of Performance	Which Organizations It Applies To	How It Relates to Disruptive Behavior
PC.5.50	"Care, treatment, and services are provided in an interdisciplinary collaborative manner."		• Ambulatory care organizations • Behavioral health care • Critical access hospitals • Home care • Hospitals • Laboratories • Long term care • Office-based surgery facilities	This standard relates to two of the important ways to diminish or reduce the incidence of disruptive behavior: effective teamwork and collaboration.
LD.1.60†	"The duties and responsibilities of the medical director are defined."	4. The medical director provides advice and input to both the administrator and the governance by doing the following: • *Monitoring employees' health status and advising the administrator on employee health policies*	• Long term care	This can relate to cases of employed staff who are disruptive by reason of impairment due to health issues.
LD.1.70	"Each leadership component contains active members who are competent, or the components have access to individuals with such competency, in the following…"	3. Training is made available to all leaders for each of the following skills: • *Identifying and resolving conflict* • Assessing processes from a system-based perspective • Working with team-based concepts • Making decisions based on evidence • *Fostering an environment of mutual respect for other team members.*	• Ambulatory care organizations • Behavioral health care • Critical access hospitals • Home care • Hospitals • Laboratories • Long term care • Office-based surgery facilities	An organization is expected to provide training for its leadership on how to identify and resolve conflict and on how to foster an environment of mutual respect for other team members; both of these concepts are important components in an effective process to manage and defuse disruptive behavior.

(continued)

* The MS chapter does not apply in all health care settings.
† The Leadership standards referred to in this table are taken from the forthcoming revised 2008 LD chapter.

Table 3-1. Joint Commission Standards and EPs Related to Disruptive Behavior, *continued*

Standard Number	Language of the Standard	Related Elements of Performance	Which Organizations It Applies To	How It Relates to Disruptive Behavior
LD.3.10	"Leaders create and maintain a culture of safety and quality throughout the organization."	4. *Leaders develop a code of conduct that includes the definition of acceptable and disruptive behaviors.* For behavioral health care organizations: *Leaders develop a code of conduct that includes the definition of acceptable and inappropriate behaviors.* 5. *Leaders create and implement a process for managing disruptive behavior.* For behavioral health care organizations: *Leaders create and implement a process for managing inappropriate behavior.*	• Ambulatory care organizations • Behavioral health care • Critical access hospitals • Home care • Hospitals • Laboratories • Long term care • Office-based surgery facilities	These EPs are a direct link to expectations of the Joint Commission related to disruptive behavior and how it is to be managed in the health care work environment.
LD.4.160	"An integrated patient safety program is implemented throughout the organization."	3. The scope of the program includes the full range of safety issues, from potential or no-harm errors (sometimes referred to as *near misses, close calls,* or *good catches*) to hazardous conditions and sentinel events, which have serious adverse outcomes. 5. There are procedures for responding to system or process failures, such as continuing to provide care, treatment, or services to those affected, containing the risk to others, and preserving factual information for subsequent analysis.	• Ambulatory care organizations • Behavioral health care • Critical access hospitals • Home care • Hospitals • Laboratories • Long term care • Office-based surgery facilities	As studies note a direct link between disruptive behavior and the increased risk to patient safety, addressing this issue has to be considered in concert with an organizationwide patient safety program.
HR.2.10	"The organization provides initial orientation."	4. As appropriate, staff orientation addresses organizationwide policies and procedures (including safety and infection control) and relevant unit, setting, or program-specific policies and procedures.	• Ambulatory care organizations • Behavioral health care • Critical access hospitals • Home care • Hospitals • Laboratories • Long term care • Office-based surgery facilities	This standard and EP relate to the kinds of orientations that should take place in an organization. As organizations are expected to have an organizationwide process and policy in place to deal with disruptive behavior, this EP provides guidance on how to disseminate that information to new staff (code of conduct).
HR.2.30	"Ongoing education, including in-services, training, and other activities, maintains and improves staff competence."	1. Staff training occurs when job responsibilities or duties change 2. Staff participate in ongoing in-services, training, or other activities to increase knowledge of work-related issues 3. Ongoing in-services and other education and training of staff are appropriate to the needs of the population(s) served and comply with law and regulation	• Ambulatory care organizations • Behavioral health care • Critical access hospitals • Home care • Hospitals • Laboratories • Long term care • Office-based surgery facilities	Some elements of effectively dealing with disruptive behavior require ongoing training and development, such as team training and communication skill building. Integrating these into ongoing training activities already under

(continued)

Table 3-1. Joint Commission Standards and EPs Related to Disruptive Behavior, *continued*

Standard Number	Language of the Standard	Related Elements of Performance	Which Organizations It Applies To	How It Relates to Disruptive Behavior
HR.2.30, *continued*		4. Ongoing in-services, training, or other staff activities emphasize specific job-related aspects of safety and infection prevention and control. 5. Ongoing in-services, training, or other staff education incorporate methods of team training, when appropriate 6. Ongoing in-services, training, and other staff education reinforce the need and ways to report unanticipated adverse events		way can expedite the process of developing those skills to help defuse and prevent disruptive behavior.
MS.4.30	"The organized medical staff defines the circumstances requiring monitoring and evaluation of a practitioner's professional performance."	2. The organized medical staff develops criteria to be used for evaluating the performance of practitioners when issues affecting the provision of safe, high-quality patient care are identified.	• Hospitals • Critical access hospitals	In cases in which an incidence of disruptive behavior by a member of the medical staff has led to a negative impact on the provision of care, treatment, and services, the process to evaluate his or her professional performance can be handled at this standard.
MS.4.80	"The medical staff implements a process to identify and manage matters of individual health for licensed independent practitioners which is separate from actions taken for disciplinary purposes."	Process design addresses the following issues: 1. Education of licensed independent practitioners and other organization staff about illness and impairment recognition issues specific to licensed independent practitioners (at-risk criteria) 2. Self-referral by a licensed independent practitioner 3. Referral by others and maintenance of informant confidentiality 4. Referral of the licensed independent practitioner to appropriate professional internal or external resources for evaluation, diagnosis, and treatment of the condition or concern 5. Maintenance of confidentiality of the licensed independent practitioner seeking referral or referred for assistance, except as limited by applicable law, ethical obligation, or when the health and safety of a patient are threatened 6. Evaluation of the credibility of a complaint, an allegation, or a concern 7. Monitoring the licensed independent practitioner and the safety of patients until the rehabilitation is complete and periodically thereafter, if required 8. Reporting to the organized medical staff leadership instances in which a licensed independent practitioner is providing unsafe treatment 9. Initiating appropriate actions when a licensed independent practitioner fails to complete the required rehabilitation program	• Hospitals • Critical access hospitals	This standard and its EPs relate directly to issues relating to physician health, such as substance abuse, emotional illness, and physical illness. As this type of impairment can lead to disruptive behavior, the two processes should be linked to each other.

Throughout the Joint Commission's standards are issues and concepts that relate to dealing with disruptive behavior. One effective way to respond quickly and effectively to disruptive behavior is to ensure that processes are already in place to help defuse such situations or prevent them from happening. This is due to the fact that the Joint Commission has framed its standards from a perspective of establishing a culture of safety and when the standards are viewed from a collective, consistent standpoint, they provide an effective blueprint for establishing that safety culture.

For Your Consideration

1. Consider Table 3-1 and take time to map out a selected EP or standard in relation to your organization and what you have in place already to defuse disruptive behavior. Use the following standard and EP to get started:
   a. LD.1.70, EP 3, "Training is made available to all leaders for each of the following skills: identifying and resolving conflict." Then consider and document what kinds of training and skill-building education you have provided to your leaders in dealing with identifying and resolving conflict. If you have provided such training, when was it last offered and to whom? How are you assessing competence and effectiveness in this area, and how are you mentoring leadership to be successful in identifying and resolving conflict?

LD.3.10: Culture of Safety and Disruptive Behavior

Probably the most challenging aspect of establishing a culture of safety is making changes in behavior and mind-set that help staff and the organization itself embrace the concept of safety in such a way that it becomes the order of the day and no longer a distant goal that organizations are working toward.

The impact and consequences of disruptive behavior are linked so intrinsically together that the Joint Commission has integrated its compliance expectations for dealing with the issue of disruptive behavior into its "culture of safety" standard:

Standard LD.3.10
Leaders create and maintain a culture of safety and quality throughout the organization.
Rationale for LD.3.10
A culture of safety and quality exists when all who work in the organization are focused on excellent performance. Leaders demonstrate their commitment to quality and set expectations for those who work in the organization. Leaders create structures, processes, and programs that allow a culture of safety and quality to flourish.

The placement of these requirements in this standard and in the "Leadership" chapter is not surprising. After all, disruptive behavior requires a leadership response, particularly as it involves eliminating it from the culture of the organization, not just dealing with incidents as they erupt. When disruptive behavior goes unchecked or is not dealt with, the impact can be so negative on the morale and culture of the organization that it impairs the organization's ability to work toward a culture of safety.

The Joint Commission explores concepts related to a culture of safety further in its introduction to the "Leadership" chapter by stating the following:

In a culture of safety and quality, all individuals are focused on maintaining excellence in performance. They accept safety and quality as personal responsibilities and work together to minimize any harm that might result from unsafe or poor quality of care, treatment, or services. Leaders create this culture by demonstrating their commitment to safety and quality and by taking actions to achieve the desired state. In this culture, one finds teamwork, open discussions of concerns about safety, and the encouragement of and reward for internal and external reporting of safety issues. Although reckless behavior and a blatant disregard for safety are not tolerated, the focus of attention is on the performance of systems and processes instead of the individual. Organizations are committed to ongoing learning and have the flexibility to accommodate changes in technology, science, and the environment.

In a presentation on patient safety, Dennis O'Leary, M.D., president of the Joint Commission, mentioned these essential qualities about establishing a culture of safety:

A culture of safety is characterized by an open atmosphere for reporting and addressing errors, and eventually by anticipating and preventing errors through careful monitoring and timely redesign of internal patient care systems. Adopting such a culture is the overarching strategy that is necessary to the realization of the full impact of other solutions to the problem, and thus the single most important strategic effort to be undertaken. But this is perhaps the most difficult goal to fully achieve. Cultural changes always require significant leadership energy and commitment. In the case of patient safety, this is even a more daunting challenge because what is actually being sought is a counter-culture to the deep-seated "blame and shame" orientation of American society. For this reason, the success of this effort depends heavily upon other key actions, such as the passage of federal "safe harbor" legislation.[2]

Complying with the Joint Commission EPs on Disruptive Behavior

As mentioned previously, the EPs that relate to disruptive behavior fall under the culture of safety standard, LD.3.10. They cover two important areas of concern:

4. Leaders develop a code of conduct that includes the definition of acceptable and disruptive behaviors.
5. Leaders create and implement a process for managing disruptive behavior.

These areas—the definition of acceptable or disruptive behaviors and developing and implementing a process—will be explored in more depth in Chapter 4; they represent the two crucial areas that leadership must have in place to address disruptive behavior: the need to develop a code of conduct that outlines what is acceptable behavior and what is disruptive behavior and the need for a process to manage disruptive behavior.

Using the Standards to Help Defuse Disruptive Behavior

The standards can be an excellent door-opener to addressing issues of disruptive behavior, particularly as they relate to staff training, orientation, and more specific areas, such as the medical staff standards. As an example, William Kragness, M.D., a consultant with Joint Commission Resources, points to MS.4.40 as an excellent way to deal with disruptive behavior in an ongoing manner. MS.4.40 states, "Ongoing professional practice evaluation information is factored into the decision to maintain existing privilege(s), to revise existing privilege(s), or

to revoke an existing privilege prior to or at the time of renewal." Kragness explains, "In the case of ongoing professional evaluation, it's an excellent process that is already in place to address or look at—in an ongoing manner—any inappropriate disruptive behavior being observed among medical staff." This approach can be fairer and more consistent and also help reinforce any training or education that may need to take place.

> ## For Your Consideration
>
> 1. Consider your own health care organization and the accreditation standards that you are surveyed under (those for hospitals, home care, laboratories, and so on) and look at Table 3-1. What other standards relate to the issue of disruptive behavior and either issues related to its impact or issues related to defusing it?
> 2. How has compliance with the standards helped your organization evolve toward a culture of safety? What steps are you taking to reach that goal?

Dealing With Disruptive Behavior

When disruptive behavior is reported in your organization, an effective and immediate response is necessary so it does not cause a chain reaction that can have a broader, negative impact on the organization itself, such as the negative effects described in Chapter 2. By dealing with the situation in a quick and effective manner, you not only send the message that the behavior is not tolerated but also can move easily to repair any damage that may have been caused by the behavior. This is analogous to how you treat a wound; it is much easier to heal a wound when it is treated as quickly as possible than when you let the wound fester, forcing sometimes a more extreme and time-consuming "cure" for the injury.

While some steps are necessary and helpful in defusing disruptive behavior, as outlined in this chapter, none of it will have a lasting, beneficial impact on an organization and its goal of establishing a culture of safety unless these processes are integrated into an overall code of conduct and process to manage disruptive behavior throughout the organization. Establishing (or reinforcing) a code of conduct and developing a broad, organizationwide process is discussed and explored further in Chapter 4. This chapter deals more specifically with what to do when a pattern or an outburst of disruptive behavior is reported or observed in your organization.

The following sections explore defusing disruptive behavior from a number of perspectives. While the attitude toward the behavior and tolerance for it should be consistent and applied in a similar fashion to any staff working within an organization (regardless of position or level of responsibility/authority), how that behavior is defused may need to vary for different staff, depending on the kind of behavior that is taking place. In addition, different individuals may need to help defuse the situation. Consider the following strategies for defusing behavior.

Getting Involved: Who Needs to Deal with Disruptive Behavior When It Happens?

Beyond the individuals directly involved with a disruptive behavior incident—the perpetrator and the victim(s)—certain key individuals in the organization can play significant roles in helping defuse disruptive behavior.

Executive leadership. In a larger organization where certain key clinical areas have an executive leader overseeing staff and development, the executive leader can and should be involved in any disruptive behavior events when they happen. Possessing the management skills necessary to help defuse disruptive behavior, executive leadership is often in the best position to help deal with the issues. They should also set the example for positive interaction with their colleagues in similar leadership positions. For example, in a hospital setting, the nurse executive and chief medical officer can demonstrate an effective and positive collaborative working relationship by working together to resolve any disruptive behavior incidents between their staff. Executive leadership can also mentor and empower the staff they work with to effectively deal with disruptive behavior when it happens to them.

In cases in which a disruptive behavior is having a pervasive and severe impact on an organization, it may also be appropriate for the chief executive officer (or comparable position) to become involved, and even the board may need to be involved. As one impact of disruptive behavior can be a negative perception of the organization by the community at large, one area where senior leadership may also have to be involved is in helping to repair any external damage caused by such an event.

Risk managers. Many larger organizations have risk management staff who can play a crucial role in helping to defuse disruptive behavior. not only is their role important in designing and establishing a policy for dealing with disruptive behavior, but they can provide valuable insight, guidance, and interventional support at the time of a disruptive behavior incident. A risk manager can be particularly helpful in gathering the necessary information and data about an event and providing guidance on what to do when intervention becomes necessary.

Risk managers can also provide—depending on their professional background and skill training—additional guidance with mentoring, mediation, or facilitation. For example, a risk manager with professional training in meditation or conflict resolution can provide crucial guidance and assistance in defusing disruptive behavior.

Department heads/staff managers. Often it is the first level of management that becomes aware of an incident of disruptive behavior. A staff member may have observed an incident, or a staff member may need to report being a victim of unacceptable behavior from a different clinician. Depending on the staff members involved and what is being reported, these first-level managers will have to respond in different ways. For example, if a nurse reports to her manager an incident of disruptive behavior from a pharmacist, then the nurse manager, in his or her investigation of the issue, will inevitably have to go to the director of pharmacy (the pharmacist's manager) and begin a formal process to consider the complaint.

Staff or peers. Often, if empowered and well-trained, staff are able to intervene at the moment that a disruptive behavior incident takes place; this can go a long way toward helping defuse the issue and restoring effective teamwork and collaboration among those involved. Sometimes all it takes is a respected peer who has observed inappropriate behavior to privately counsel the perpetrator as to why their behavior is unacceptable, and the damage can be quickly repaired. For example, if a physician observes one of his or her colleagues acting disruptively toward other staff, it may be effective and helpful if that physician—a peer—takes a moment to privately pull that other physician aside to talk about what happened and help counsel them on remedying the situation (making an apology, using more effective means to communicate a concern, using more appropriate channels to share concerns with organization leadership, and so on).

Staff psychologists or psychiatrists. Some organizations have on staff—typically for other reasons related to the type of care, treatment, or services that they provide—psychologists or psychiatrists. Depending on the kind of disruptive behavior and its impact, it can be beneficial to engage such a professional in helping to defuse an incidence of disruptive behavior. Because effectively defusing disruptive behavior requires a behavioral shift in the perpetrator, a trained professional can make a big difference in helping staff overcome the behaviors that make them act out disruptively or help staff who have been victims of abuse. For organizations without such a resource on staff, other therapeutic services, such as employee assistance programs or outside psychologists or psychiatrists, might be an option.

Employee wellness committees, nurse wellness committees, physician health/wellness committees. With the advent of staff health issues—from injuries in the workplace to substance or alcohol abuse and emotional health—some organizations have established "wellness committees" to deal with any health issues that may impact staff. Such a committee can also play an important role in helping to deal with disruptive behavior. When studying the cause of disruptive behavior (as explored in Chapter 2), it has been found that some causes of disruptive behavior are directly related to health—substance and alcohol abuse, emotional illness, personality disorders, physical illnesses, personal problems, and so on. These committees typically have in place processes to help staff effectively.

External organizations, intervention programs, mediation experts. At times it can be helpful to draw from external sources to assist with defusing disruptive behavior. Some professional organizations that your health care organization is already affiliated with may offer guidance or information on dealing with disruptive behavior. In addition, there may be some external associations or organizations that specialize in assisting health care organizations in dealing with disruptive behavior. In looking for such external sources, it may be worth considering whether anyone has been brought in in the past or if other organizations can suggest individuals or organizations.

The following case study describes how Vanderbilt University Hospital has used the wellness committee approach and dedicated professional staff (and a treatment program) to help its staff deal with any health issues.

CASE STUDY 3-1
WORKERS GET HELP FOR DRUGS, ALCOHOL, AND OTHER IMPAIRMENTS
Vanderbilt University Hospital Runs Successful Treatment Program

Case Study at a Glance

Vanderbilt University Medical Center is an 800-bed tertiary care hospital that comprises Vanderbilt School of Medicine and the Vanderbilt School of Nursing. Vanderbilt Clinic had more than 698,900 patient visits during 2003, and Vanderbilt Hospital admitted more than 33,800 patients.

Main challenge: Help physicians, nurses, faculty, and staff address issues of drug and alcohol abuse and mental health problems

Issues: Get help for clinical staff plus medical school faculty and staff

Joint Commission standards: Standard MS.4.80 requires all accredited hospitals and medical practices to have in place a process that addresses health issues of licensed independent practitioners in a way that is separate from discipline.

Solutions: Vanderbilt's Work/Life Connections program helps impaired workers get evaluated, diagnosed, and referred for treatment.

Outcome: More than 95% of self-referrals and mandatory referrals complete Vanderbilt's three-year program.

By 1998, it had become apparent that the health of clinicians and others on the staff of Vanderbilt Hospital needed attention. In the years preceding, the careers of eight physicians had been cut short by tragedy. Four physicians died; two were suicides, one died from domestic violence, and one died from an indeterminate cause. Four other incidents, including three involving sexual misconduct, also came to the attention of Mary Yarbrough, M.D., M.P.H., director of Health and Wellness at Vanderbilt University and director of the Vanderbilt Center for Occupational and Environmental Medicine.

In response, members of the Vanderbilt Medical Board agreed to initiate a physician wellness program focused on prevention of impairment and education of impaired physicians, whether from mental health issues or drug or alcohol abuse. The Vanderbilt program preceded the Joint Commission standard on licensed independent practitioner wellness but matched it closely and included many of the same components specified in standard MS.4.80—education, diagnosis, treatment, evaluation, reporting, monitoring, prevention, and referral.

Dr. Yarbrough describes the programs—the Physician Wellness Program and the Nursing Wellness Program—as subsets of Vanderbilt's Work/Life Connections employee assistance program (EAP). "Our programs cover not just problems with alcohol and drugs but all mental health concerns, and the majority of cases are self-referrals," says Yarbrough. When impaired medical professionals enter the Vanderbilt program as either self-referrals or mandatory referrals, they are evaluated, diagnosed, and allowed to choose from among three of the community's best providers with experience in physician impairment. The Vanderbilt Center works with the physicians' insurance companies and assigns a staff psychiatrist as well as a social worker who functions as a case manager until the physician recovers and/or the case is closed.

"We help them identify whatever resource they need," says Yarbrough. "We follow them throughout the program, and if they're mandatory referrals, we follow them for at least six months afterward. If they're getting help for an addiction, we might follow them for as long as three years." Yarbrough points out that if a physician disagrees with the need for treatment, as is often the case with disruptive behavior, Vanderbilt may send the person elsewhere for an independent evaluation. "The main thing," says Yarbrough, "is to get a diagnosis and a treatment plan."

In addition to the physician and nursing wellness programs, Vanderbilt also offers help to members of its staff and faculty. The priority in every case is patient safety," says Yarbrough. "We ask a number of questions: Is it safe for this person to work? Are they a threat to themselves or anyone else? Do they need any accommodations for their impairment?" Yarbrough deals with organizational issues such as Why is this referral mandatory? Are there any disciplinary issues? If so, have they been dealt with in the appropriate format? Are there any legal issues or employee discrimination or employee relations issues? Yarbrough also collaborates with other department heads to make sure these things are handled according to the Vanderbilt policy. "With mandatory referrals, we bring in the physician and explain how the program works, what is considered confidential, and when information is released," says Yarbrough. A clinician must sign a release for any information that is distributed about that person unless required by law or the patient is a threat to patient safety. All this is on a strictly need-to-know basis. Meanwhile, Vanderbilt psychiatrists and social workers continue dealing with the clinical components of the person's recovery, such as What is the diagnosis and treatment plan? Is it safe for the person to practice? Are there any restrictions to his or her practicing? Is any monitoring needed in the workplace?

Changing Parameters

When Vanderbilt launched its program six years ago, it was helping no more than eight people a year. Most of them had already begun treatment for drug and alcohol problems and were coming to the Work/Life Connections EAP for drug screenings. Since then, the number of people treated in the program has increased substantially. Between April 2005 and January 2006, Vanderbilt's Physician Wellness Program received 120 referrals, of which 90% were self-referrals. Only 10% were for drug and/or alcohol addiction; the remaining referrals were for other issues.

Self-medication with a prescription drug is often unmasked in the course of working with other behavioral health conditions. Yarbrough points out that depression and other psychological problems are the major problem these days, accounting for 40% of referrals. "There is a whole other group whose primary problem might not be addiction, but in the course of the recovery, they'll be treated for that as well." Thanks to extensive experience, the professionals who run the Work/Life Connections program are able to pick up on problems early and deal with them before they become acute and involve disciplinary issues. "The majority of self-referrals are simply unhappy," says Yarbrough, "and they want help for their illness."

Areas of Concern

According to Yarbrough, anesthesiology is an area of concern because of easy access to prescription drugs. "There's also the abuse of alcohol across the board," she continues. Yarbrough has found that, with physicians, unless they're very much out of control, their impairment can be quite difficult to detect. It may come down to a dramatic event in the workplace, and sometimes several incidents have happened well before that. "The more referrals we get, the earlier we're likely to pick up on alcohol and drug addiction," says Yarbrough.

Of the 120 people who are treated in a year, about 40% are seen for psychological problems; 20% are relational and family issues; 30% come to deal with workplace behavior, such as being disruptive or acting out at work; about 10% are seen for alcohol and drug problems; and the remainder are considered "other." To care for the health care providers, Vanderbilt has three psychiatrists who work part time, one psychologist, four social workers, and a nurse practitioner who works with the Nursing Wellness Program.

Issues Addressed by Vanderbilt's Work/Life Connections Program

- Stress/emotional issues
- Depression/grief/loss
- Family/marital conflicts
- Interpersonal concerns
- Divorce adjustment
- Domestic violence
- Alcohol/substance abuse
- Relationship issues
- Critical incident stress management

As noted, the Vanderbilt program has expanded beyond physicians to cover members of the faculty, the nursing staff, and also the postdoctoral population at the medical center. Yarbrough reports that the faculty and staff members served by Vanderbilt's Physician Wellness Program number about 2,500—mostly clinical and including residents. "We're finding increasing numbers of special needs among professionals," she reports, "because of their licensure requirements and because they're doing clinical work involving patient safety issues. The process is far more complicated when it involves licensure."

Yarbrough attributes the credit for the program's success to the Vanderbilt medical staff. "The leadership here has been quite supportive. They want to reduce stress and burnout among physicians. Instead of 'catching' and 'punishing' impaired clinicians, they understand these behavioral mental health and substance-related conditions to be diseases and, as such, to require appropriate diagnosis, treatment, and follow-up. With patient safety as the number-one priority, the issue is, how can we help the physicians?"

The message of the Vanderbilt program is that, like everyone else, clinicians have mental health and substance abuse problems. The majority of self-referrals respond well to appropriate referral for counseling and treatment. Those who go to treatment for addiction or who are especially disruptive must sign a contract with multiple components. They must also check in periodically with the Vanderbilt program, where they're subject to random drug screenings. Those with addictions must also enter into an agreement with the state of Tennessee. "When they get their health back, and their disease is in remission," says Yarbrough, "we continue to support their recovery and help them get back to work. They have a big financial, intellectual, and emotional investment in their professional capability. And more than 95% of the referrals who require an agreement make it through our three-year program."

Source: Originally printed in *Environment of Care News*, June 2006, Volume 9, Issue 6.

Figure 3-1, page 44, provides an example of a behavior report form that can be used.

For Your Consideration

1. In the Vanderbilt case study, what are some elements of the program that you can point to that seem particularly effective or germane to the issue of disruptive behavior?

2. Considering your organization's data, what kind of issues have you faced in relation to health issues? Have you had any substance or alcohol abuse issues? If you have, how have you dealt with them?

3. In considering your own organization, what kind of program should you design for staff health issues? Or, if you have a program in place already, how does it compare to the one described in the case study and what, if any, changes would you want to make to improve your program?

Interventional Steps: Defusing Disruptive Behavior

As illustrated in the Vanderbilt case study, the approach to defusing disruptive behavior can differ depending on the situation and who needs to be involved in helping to deal with it. There are also a number of steps that can be taken to help deal with the variety of situations that can emerge from disruptive behavior, but most experts agree that the following must be part of the overall process: do it sooner rather than later; interview staff and gather as much background information as possible; when interviewing the staff member involved, always keep in mind that the behavior could be pointing to a systems issue (not excusing the behavior, how-ever); always keep a paper trail; and maintain confidentiality. The following steps illustrate some of the key elements that must be in place to help defuse a disruptive situation.

Step 1: Provide a Reporting Process

An organization needs to ensure that it has in place a process to report a complaint or concern and that this process is communicated to staff. Staff will typically inform their direct manager or staff leader when there is a problem. It is also possible that an inappropriate event was observed by many staff members and that an observer has reported it. This reporting process should be confidential, but it should be made clear to the person reporting a specific incident that when the investigation process begins, the staff member being reported may well learn of the report and investigation (and thereby at least identify the person the event or events that led to the complaint).

Step 2: Investigate the Issue Thoroughly and Rapidly

Once a report has been submitted, it is important for the matter to be investigated thoroughly and rapidly. As challenging as it can be to have to approach a staff member about a report of his or her disruptive behavior, the sooner the issue is dealt with, the easier it is for everyone involved. The investigation may require speaking confidentially to other staff and speaking directly to the people involved in the situation. The most important thing to keep in mind at this stage is to avoid a confrontational style. Many times, during the initial interview and discussion process, resolutions can emerge. The disruptive staff member may become immediately apologetic and take steps to rectify the situation with the person he or she has hurt. Approaching the disruptive staff member in too confrontational a tone could unnecessarily escalate the process when a solution might be readily available.

Also, when interviewing the person who was disruptive, it can be very helpful to ask what, if any, circumstances led the person to have such an inappropriate reaction. Was there a systems issue? Did something happen? Are there issues that the staff member has with the organization that need to be considered or addressed? It can be helpful at that time to remind the staff member that there are other and more appropriate ways to address concerns with the organization and that any kind of disruptive behavior is an unacceptable method to get any message across.

It is also important to hear the full story from the person on the receiving end of the disruptive behavior. It can be extremely helpful to that person to feel heard and respected because his or her own sense of personal well-being may have been affected by the experience. It is also good to interview the person filing the complaint so that he or she knows an appropriate process is under way to address their concerns. All too often a staff member who has been on the receiving end of disruptive behavior will complain to a third party and not want to communicate any concerns through appropriate channels or directly to the person who was disruptive, and this ends up adding to the already damaged work environment and could affect the situation negatively.

Figure 3-1. Sample Behavior Report Form

Staff Involved:		Event Location:	
Event Date:	Event Time:	Name of Submitter:	
Location (room no., department):		Record No.:	Account No.:

Submitter's Description of Inappropriate Behavior Events: *(objective, factual account to include behaviors witnessed, precipitating circumstances, and any action taken to remedy situation)*

Analysis/Resolution:

Step 3: Intervene with a Plan of Action and Follow Through

When the full situation has been investigated and considered from a variety of perspectives, it is important to make a plan and take action. This can involve preparing a plan of action for the staff member to follow based on the disruptive behavior and its causes. It is also helpful, if the staff member is cooperative, to work out the plan with the staff member him- or herself. For example, in the case of disruptive behavior that results from alcohol abuse, the plan of action may be referring the staff member to a treatment program or a wellness program. Or it may be asking the staff member to undergo an anger management class or to improve their communication skills.

Whatever the plan, it is extremely important to follow through and monitor progress because this is often where actual changed behavior will take hold. It is also important to set a realistic and reachable time frame for compliance with the action plan. The plan should include regular check-ins to ensure that the steps laid

out are being followed or, if adjustments need to be made, that they are written into the formal plan.

In their research on practice compliance programs, Olver and West suggest that the following elements be a part of any solution or plan that is created:

- Goal
- Benchmark
- Objectives
- Monitoring
- Consequence clause[2]

The plan should include a goal, which is to eliminate problematic behavior and actions of the person involved. The benchmark is the starting mark, the point where the action became a problem and was identified. By quantifying the problem into a measure set of data, following the remaining essentials of the solution is achievable. The objectives list what must be done to eliminate the problem and generate acceptable behavior by a set date (also part of the plan). Monitoring involves tracking the subject's subsequent behavior relevant to the problem that originated the plan. Finally, the consequence clause refers to a document that is written—which the subject signs and agrees to—and states that the problem is understood, there is agreement to follow the steps to address it, and the signer accepts any consequences that may be noted in the event that the problem is not rectified.[3]

Also keep in mind the importance of positive encouragement and feedback along the way. Change is never simple, and in many of these cases, a challenging and troubling situation has brought the offending staff member and leadership to this point. Being willing and able to take the necessary steps to make improvements and change one's personal behavior takes courage and effort; this should be acknowledged and encouraged throughout.

Any plan to defuse disruptive behavior needs to include and take into consideration the whole work environment when working to deal with the issue. Disruptive behavior can and does have a negative impact on staff, even those who are not directly involved in an incident or a series of incidents. Any plan needs to take into consideration the health and well-being of all those involved, even if they are involved indirectly. This can include allowing staff—if they desire it—an opportunity to discuss and share their thoughts and concerns and, if necessary, providing additional therapy or mediation services to help staff move past any issues that may prevent the team working together well. All discussions and actions on this part should remain confidential.

Step 4: Follow-up and Acknowledgment
In the best-case scenario, the aforementioned steps are successfully followed, and a staff member who was displaying disruptive behavior has found correct channels through which to address his or her behavior and has taken effective steps to prevent the behavior from recurring. The organization has helped one of its valued staff members address his or her unacceptable behavior, and the organization is not impaired by any impact to staff morale or patient safety. On the other hand, in a realistic scenario, there may be more failures than successes, but those successes need to be celebrated as well. Overcoming disruptive behavior takes time and consistent effort.

This kind of success needs to be acknowledged. Successfully and meaningfully modifying or improving behavior requires great will on the part of the individual, and it is no easy task. Achieving such a significant milestone should be celebrated

and acknowledged. This kind of success resonates with the organization as well. Not only do staff feel empowered by feeling that their needs and concerns are heard and acknowledged, they realize that the organization takes its commitment to establishing a patient-safe environment seriously. These kinds of responses and their successes go a long way toward helping cement that evolution toward a culture of safety.

In addition, this kind of action sends a clear message: The behavior is what needs to be rectified, not the individual. Working on a plan to eliminate a staff member's disruptive behavior and not focusing on eliminating the staff member him- or herself says to the organization that people are valuable—but their behavior can sometimes be out of sync with the culture of the organization. All too often, people who are under the "cloud" of a corrective process feel like they are no longer wanted at the organization, and they may feel demoralized to the point of leaving the organization entirely.

Step 5: Contingency Plans
Unfortunately, there are times when a plan does not succeed, and the "consequence clause" needs to be put into action. Depending on the situation and what was determined when the original plan was put in place, it is important to carry out whatever consequence was decided at that time or, if warranted, to make a determination for another alternative. For example, consider the case of a physician who is not complying with a substance abuse treatment program; year-long efforts to help her rehabilitate were unsuccessful. In the original plan, the consequence clause may have stated that her privileges may be suspended, or there might be financial sanctions if the physician fails to comply with the plan of action as agreed. The consequence may escalate actions, too, for example, with a requirement in place for the physician to attend a residential treatment program for professionals.

It is not always possible to see success with every effort to defuse disruptive behavior. There are cases in which the staff member is unwilling or unable to make the appropriate changes in behavior so that he or she can continue to work in the organization. In those cases, steps must be in place (as explored in more depth in Chapter 4) to terminate employment or the working relationship, depending on how the staff member interacts with the organization.

The previously discussed steps lay out a possible approach to dealing with the problem of defusing disruptive behavior. The following scenario illustrates how those steps might be carried out.

Ways to Defuse Disruptive Behavior:

Dealing with a Problem Physician

Over the past year, the ambulatory surgical center's chief medical officer (CMO) had received more than a dozen complaints from surgical nurses, surgical technicians, and anesthesiologists about Dr. Tom Baxter's ongoing disruptive behavior in the OR. The reports noted such things as "verbal abuse," "extensive criticism," "threat of punishment or punitive response," and "perfectionism gone awry." On four previous occasions, the CMO had spoken to Dr. Baxter to discuss more effective ways to explore any issues that may be causing the behavior. Each time Dr. Baxter had expressed remorse over his behavior but would always point to certain issues that seemed to be triggers for him.

After the latest report, the nurse manager told the CMO that she believed the nurse who had filed it was preparing to find a new position with a different surgical center due to her dissatisfaction with how the surgeon's behavior seemed to be enabled and her frustration with the abuse she felt while trying to do her job. She felt sure, her report noted, "that one of these days, we're going to make a big mistake in a surgery because we'll be so stressed out by how he treats us."

The CMO didn't delay. When he saw Dr. Baxter in the hall the next day, he asked if they could make some time to talk. Dr. Baxter nodded and said he would come by after surgery. Two hours later, Dr. Baxter walked into the CMO's office. The CMO explained the report and how that, combined with the previous record of complaints, forced him to need to investigate the issue and come up with a plan of action. Dr. Baxter seemed perplexed, and his response supported that observation. "You know, it's easy to point the finger at me, just because I'm direct and don't mince words."

The CMO proceeded with an investigation and gathered any data and documentation he could find. His research found that Dr. Baxter had been a successful surgeon who generated a high amount of revenue. But he also found that Dr. Baxter was repeatedly reported for disruptive behavior, and he even noted a few times when nurses had requested not to be assigned to his cases. The CMO then interviewed the nurse who filed the report. Carrie was a highly skilled OR nurse with a long tenure at the surgical center, and was not someone who typically complained. But in her interview with the CMO, she said that she had had enough. "That day in the OR, he threatened to 'slap me silly' because I didn't hand him an instrument fast enough. He makes everyone nervous and uncomfortable. We're more prone to snap at each other as a result. I have seen the younger nurses hesitate more around him." The CMO also spoke, confidentially, with other staff members about what had happened, and he get a more complete picture.

After gathering more information, he met with Dr. Baxter again and shared his findings. At first Dr. Baxter was surprised by how his style of communicating was viewed as disruptive. However, after discussing the issue in more depth and after the CMO pointed to the negative impact his actions and behavior were having on not only the staff around him but on the organization itself, Dr. Baxter seemed more open to discussing the issue. The CMO stated that he knew that Dr. Baxter was committed to excellence and that his work was not in question, but his methods were not a fit for the organization.

Once the CMO was able to convey to the surgeon the message that his behavior was actually making matters worse, Dr. Baxter agreed to make some adjustments. The CMO then devised a plan that they both agreed to. The first step was for the surgeon to use more productive and less abrasive communication. To help him, the CMO gave him examples of ways to communicate and also arranged for him to work with a leadership consultant on a one-on-one basis to improve his teamwork and communication skills.

The CMO and Dr. Baxter would meet monthly to discuss progress. Although Dr. Baxter still had times when he was more abrupt than was ideal, his communication skills and approach improved dramatically. Dr. Baxter was more aware of the interpersonal impact he was having on those around him and, as a result, curbed his disruptive behavior.

For Your Consideration

1. In any interventions that you have been involved in, what steps did you take to defuse the situation? What lessons did you learn? How many successful interventions have you had and how many have resulted in termination?
2. What training do you or your leadership colleagues have in defusing disruptive behavior? What training do you feel you need?

In the following case study, Ron May, M.D., vice president of Medical Affairs at Craven Medical Center, shares his perspective and experiences with disruptive physician behavior and how he works to defuse any reported situations.

CASE STUDY 3-2
LEADING AT THE FRONTLINE:
DISRUPTIVE PHYSICIAN BEHAVIOR
IN A MIDSIZE HOSPITAL

Case Study at a Glance

Name: Craven Regional Medical Center

Location: New Bern, North Carolina

Organization information: Craven Regional Medical Center is a 313-bed, full-service facility that provides a wide range of inpatient services, such as medical/surgical care, neurosurgical care, intensive and intermediate care, women's care, pediatric care, and cancer care. It provides services to 15,000 inpatients annually.

Purpose: Craven Regional Medical Center provides mentoring and direct intervention for its medical staff when a report of disruptive behavior is filed.

"We have had incidences of disruptive physician behavior at our hospital," notes Ron May, M.D., F.A.C.H.E., F.A.A.P., C.P.E., vice president for Medical Affairs at

Craven Medical Center in New Bern, North Carolina. "But it has been relatively infrequent when I've had to become formally involved in my capacity as vice president for Medical Affairs." May estimates that his 313-bed hospital receives formal reports of a disruptive physician about once a year. He also notes that there are additional incidents that are either resolved informally or are isolated. "Often if a physician is disruptive and a colleague is aware of it, that colleague may intervene by privately discussing the issue with the physician to help him or her address the disruptive behavior," May notes. May has also observed that sometimes the staff member who was on the receiving end of the disruptive behavior addresses the issue at the time of the incident, though that takes place very infrequently. He also acknowledges that some cases are just not formally reported and can go left unchecked for a while.

"In order to begin the formal process to address disruptive behavior, a report has to be made to a manager, and then it comes to me to facilitate bringing it to the attention of the Medical Executive Committee," May explains. May has found that those complaints are typically based in fact. "For a staff member to formally report the process means that it has become uncomfortable enough for them to be willing to take it to that next level." May will then sit down with the physician privately to discuss what happened from his or her perspective and to share the complaint. "I prefer to keep the process as collegial and positive as possible, but I am direct in addressing what happened and talking about why the behavior is unacceptable," May notes. He also acknowledges that one cannot sugar coat the behavior or what took place. "It's not a comfortable experience to have to tell someone that their behavior has been unacceptable—but you have to address it quickly and consistently. Your goal is to critique not the person but the behavior."

May has had cases in which a physician is immediately apologetic for his or her behavior and makes an immediate effort to repair any damage caused. Sometimes the disruptive behavior can manifest itself in unexpected ways. May recounted an example: "We had a physician—a surgeon—who had a particularly large physique and an at-times intimidating demeanor.

He was prone to outbursts of anger or frustration that were most likely amplified by his size. This was actually causing staff to feel unsafe and threatened. After receiving reported incidences of this behavior, I sat down with him to discuss what was happening. I explained how his particular style of communicating was having a negative impact on staff and care delivery. This surgeon did not realize the impact of his behavior and was immediately apologetic. We did not receive any other reported concerns about this surgeon after this incident."

Unfortunately, not all cases of disruptive behavior can be resolved so quickly. "We do have those physicians who do not seem to appreciate how their disruptive behavior is an unacceptable means by which to get a message across or to share a concern," May continues. In cases in which a physician is not willing to immediately improve his or her behavior, the physician will usually be referred to their state's physician's health program (PHP). "The program deals with a wide variety of behavior issues, from impairment to inappropriate behavior, and we have seen success from participating in such a program."

Overall, May suggests that organizations respond quickly and effectively to any report of disruptive behavior, noting that work must be done to address and eliminate the unacceptable behavior, not the individual. In addition, he often reminds physicians that if they want to work effectively with the rest of the care team, it's in their best interest to communicate well, be civil, and collaborate with all staff for the benefit of the patient.

The Role of the Defuser
Defusing disruptive behavior requires patience, responsiveness, and focus. It is never an easy job to address an issue that speaks to someone's behavior and, even, personality. Dealing with disruptive behavior effectively takes time, commitment, and a consistent approach. It requires training and good communication skills. Above all, it requires a focus on the behavior and not on the person. Some common pitfalls or mistakes have been made in the past when attempting to defuse disruptive behavior; leaders need to keep them in mind when navigating this task.

Sidebar 3-1, page 49, lists a number of common mistakes made in managing disruptive behavior. While this list speaks specifically to certain kinds of staff, such as physicians, the sidebar is intended to provide guidance on pitfalls for organizations to try to avoid while dealing with disruptive behavior in all types of staff in a health care organization.

Defusing Disruptive Behavior: Staff Response
It is never easy for a staff member to deal with disruptive behavior, but in order to ensure a safe, well-functioning work environment, such behavior should not be tolerated. As such, there are times when a staff member may find him- or herself either needing to report an incident of disruptive behavior or having to deal with it directly. Staff should have means of reporting any concerns or experiences to their managers and should never feel alone in their response to the issue. There are times, however, when a direct response can be helpful. The following are some suggestions on how staff who are on the receiving end of disruptive behavior can deal with it:

- **Step 1: Reacting in the Moment**
  Ending disruptive behavior requires both long- and short-term action. Reacting productively and protectively in the moment is difficult, says Cheryl Johnson, president of the United American Nurses, AFL-CIO. She suggests that staff ask themselves a few pertinent questions at the time of the incident: "What effect does this incident have on patient care?" and "What effect does this incident have on me?" Asking these questions helps the staff member remove him- or herself and the patient from the situation and see what risk may still remain. Johnson offers the following suggestions for swift, appropriate action, depending on the answers to the questions:
  - React immediately with a response that is appropriate to the situation, by saying something to the effect of "I can't answer you while you are yelling. If you lower your voice, I'll respond."
  - Redirect the focus onto the patient's needs to depersonalize the issue.
  - Move the conflict away from the patient care areas. If you feel threatened, move closer to other staff.
  - If you witness verbal abuse, call out a signal to let your coworkers know to stand by silently and act as witnesses to the abuse. Witnesses can serve an important purpose of corroborating the events that have transpired, but some abusers will modify their behavior if others are present.

Sidebar 3-1
Common Errors in Managing Problem Behaviors

1. **Hoping the problem will work itself out without any active effort.** "Let's just wait a while to see what happens; maybe it'll work itself out." Do not act prematurely, but once you are sure a staff member is being disruptive, act immediately.
2. **Not taking the first step.** Before you do anything else, determine the cause of the disruptive behavior. Like diabetes, depression, and dementia, disruptive behavior is a descriptive catchall term. Sudden outbursts of uncontrollable anger can be due to a brain tumor. They can also be caused by high-liability insurance premiums or a heavy-handed executive management style. Design strategies to deal with the causes of disruptive behavior.
3. **Trying to prove that the disruptive staff member is incompetent.** When the problem is substandard clinical performance, collect data about clinical practice. When the problem is disruptive behavior, carefully document the time and details of incidents judged to be disruptive. There is a difference between the two, and it may not be possible or advisable to try to link the two together.
4. **Inadvertently using pejorative language when trying to deal with the behavior.** Resolving an issue can be especially difficult if the language used to deal with the problem becomes a barrier in and of itself. For example, saying something like "Look, Doc, we're just trying to help you here" could be seen as pejorative and inflame an already tense situation. For many physicians, for example, "Doc" is a disrespectful term.
5. **Going to the medical staff bylaws or staff guidelines/policies and/or using legal means to deal with the problem.** While a disruptive person may eventually leave you no choice but to impose administrative and legal remedies, the first step in dealing with disruptive behavior should be constructive confrontation.
6. **Giving certain kinds of staff special treatment.** "Yes, I know he pushed one of the nurses the other day in the OR, but he's one of our best surgeons." If some organization employees or staff are given wide latitude and tolerance for types of disruptive behavior, while others are immediately penalized (and even terminated) for the same, it can create a demoralizing work environment that sends the message that some staff are "above the law." It also communicates to colleagues of the staff who get special treatment that they are also afforded the same privilege, which can perpetuate the broader acceptance of disruptive behavior.
7. **Trying to conceal the problem from the board.** While the presence of a disruptive staff member in the organization may not reflect negatively on performance, hiding information from the board can. Advise the board about the problem as soon as possible, before they learn about the problem from somewhere else.
8. **Bringing in external consultants and turning the whole matter over to them.** It may be necessary to look outside the organization for skills and expertise to help assess, advise on, resolve, and solve the problem, but this must be combined with leadership support and active involvement. Outside resources may be a great help in solving a problem, but the driving force and leadership to really resolve the issues must come from within the organization.
9. **Believing that disruptive behavior is forever.** It is possible that some staff members' behaviors or actions are so egregious or damaging that it is not suitable or possible for them to practice or work at the organization again. But for the most part, many staff members can work through their issues and successfully remain on staff and viable to the organization. An organization's policy and approach to disruptive behavior should take into consideration reinstatement, rehabilitation, and reintegration into the work environment. It should also acknowledge when behavior is overcome and improved upon.

• **Step 2: Following Up, Taking Systemic Action**

Once you and the patient are away from the threat, reporting the incident is important. Johnson notes that too often, abused staff will do nothing and hope that it does not happen again. By not acting, the person who is disruptive gets the nonverbalized message that it is okay to act that way because no one did anything to address it. The reporting process should involve a way to submit a written report. Include as many details as possible. In fact, keeping a personal document of as many specific details as possible (who, what, when, where, how) can be helpful in keeping the facts and details straight. Johnson also notes that if the staff member is part of a union (such as the United American Nurses, AFL-CIO), a report should also be submitted to the union.

• **Step 3: Insisting on a Response**

An abusive situation does not end once reports are submitted. For organizations with processes in place to deal with the behavior, what typically follows are interviews and additional investigations. Don't let the ball drop; it is important to feel that the process is moving ahead. Discussing the issue with your manager can help keep you updated on progress and aware of any development, as appropriate.[4] An organization with a consistent and well-framed process in place will not let the ball drop and will work closely with those involved to work beyond the issues to ensure that a civil work environment is in place.

Defusing disruptive behavior is not a simple task, but it is manageable when a consistent, well-thought-out, decisive, and comprehensive process is in place to deal with it. Effectively defusing disruptive behavior ensures that its negative impact on an organization's culture does not go unchecked and is resolved before it can have a lasting effect.

It is essential to have the necessary skills and capability to effectively deal with and defuse disruptive behavior as it happens. However, another important step is to have in place systems and processes that provide important guidance and information on how an organization expects its staff and employees to behave toward each other and also shares what will happen in the advent of disruptive behavior. Establishing policies and procedures to deal with disruptive behavior is explored in more depth in Chapter 4.

References

1. Gallup D.G.: The disruptive physician: Myth of reality. *Am J Obstet Gynecol* 195(2):543–546, 2006.
2. O'Leary D.: "Patient Safety: Instilling Hospitals with a Culture of Continuous Improvement." Testimony before the Senate Committee on Governmental Affairs, June 11, 2003.
3. Olver J., West D.: Practice compliance programs: Reducing therapeutic misadventures and adverse outcomes. *J Med Pract Manage* 188:187–193, Jan./Feb. 2000.
4. Johnson C.L., DeMass Martin S., Markle-Elder S.: Stopping verbal abuse in the workplace. *Am J Nurs* 107(4):32–34, 2007.

Chapter 4

Implementing a Zero-Tolerance Policy

In this chapter: Every health care organization should have a zero-tolerance policy for staff who behave disruptively. This chapter gives tips on shaping and implementing an effective disruptive behavior policy and includes examples of policies and procedures from health care organizations working to effectively implement a zero-tolerance policy.

Earlier chapters have identified what disruptive behavior is, how it is carried out, who typically does it, what causes it, and its impact. In addition, compliance expectations relating to disruptive behavior and methods to defuse the behavior have also been explored. This chapter looks at how to develop and implement a process that promulgates a zero-tolerance policy for disruptive behavior. It also looks at ways to foster the organizationwide skills that are necessary to sustain and nurture a work environment that is free of disruptive behavior.

The imperative to ensure that environments are free from disruptive behavior has never been stronger. Many have determined that it's not enough to verbalize a commitment to defusing and preventing disruptive behavior in the work environment; this commitment has to be paired with an organizationwide and consistent process in the form of policies, a code of conduct, and a mapped-out process. In addition, training and education must be made available to help foster the important components of a disruptive behavior–free work environment, particularly teamwork, collaboration, and effective communication.

Implementing a Zero-Tolerance Policy for Disruptive Behavior Organizationwide

There is no excuse for disruptive behavior, and an organization should take pains to ensure that its policies and procedures mirror that point of view. A zero-tolerance policy should state that there is no tolerance—in any capacity—for disruptive behavior in the organization by any staff member in the work environment. This includes full-time staff, medical staff with privileges, and temporary or contracted staff. Any staff member—no matter how little they may interact with the work environment—can have a negative (or, hopefully, positive) impact on those around him or her. Part of ensuring that staff abide by and follow a zero-tolerance policy is to put in place an organizationwide code of conduct and ensure that staff are aware of it and agree to abide by it.

An Organizationwide Code of Conduct for Acceptable and Disruptive Behaviors

In its new elements of performance (EPs) related to disruptive behavior, The Joint Commission requires that health care organizations create a code of conduct for acceptable and disruptive behaviors (LD.3.10, EP 5). The exact language and content of this code are up to the organization itself and what needs to be reinforced, but this code must be in place to comply with this EP. In the past, a code of conduct may have been written for the medical staff only. Or, a code of conduct may have existed in different places in an organization's policies and procedures, but it was enforced and communicated in an inconsistent manner. The new EP tells organizations that leaders must establish a code and that it must be organizationwide.

The code need not be complex. It could simply be a statement that reads, "All individuals in this organization are entitled to be treated with respect, courtesy, and dignity, and will not be treated in a manner that impairs their safety, productivity, well-being, or self-worth in the organization."[1]

Experts provide the following guidance on what concepts should be included in a code, and a number of examples in this chapter (*see* Figures 4-1, 4-2, and 4-3 on pages 59–68) share how other organizations have framed the language of their own codes of conduct. It is important, however, to keep in mind that the guidance and examples are guidance and examples, and organization leaders need to ensure that their code fits the needs and expectations of their own organization and meets and complements their goals of establishing and sustaining a culture of safety. Chapter 1 includes a list of disruptive behaviors that can be included in a code of conduct to help identify unacceptable behaviors.

One way to determine what should be in the code of conduct is to involve as wide and varied a spectrum of staff and perspectives as possible. A few approaches can be considered to achieve that goal: using a team-based approach to designing and drafting the code, having a group discussion (at staff meetings, for example) to brainstorm on the code, or surveying staff on the qualities and elements they value in the workplace that should be in the code. Using a strategy of including as many perspectives as possible can also help an organization ensure that as many staff as possible are engaged in supporting the code and its establishment. People tend to be more invested in supporting an idea if they feel a sense of ownership in its success.

In developing the code of conduct it is important to determine what you *do and do not* want to see in a work environment. In any work environment, there are some common truths to the ways that most believe their coworkers (and themselves) should behave. Some qualities could include the following:
- Effective teamwork and collaboration
- Supportive work environment
- Open communication
- Civility
- Encouragement
- Mutual respect
- Honesty
- Cooperation

There is also a series of behaviors that many will agree coworkers should *refrain* from demonstrating in the work environment, which could include the following:
- Sexual innuendo, abuse, or harassment
- Racism, sexism, or ethic slurs
- Being violent or threatening violence
- Exhibiting an intimidating manner
- Using foul language, shouting, or being rude
- Being openly critical of staff in front of others
- Threatening retribution or litigation

Through a process of brainstorming and storytelling, you can learn about what other issues are prevalent and have a negative impact on the work environment and patient safety. See Figure 4-1 on pages 59–64 for an example of a code of conduct established for medical staff.

In Sidebar 4-1 on page 53, John-Henry Pfifferling, Ph.D., director of the Center for Professional Well-Being, delineates the descriptors for professional behaviors (appropriate code of conduct) and descriptors of unprofessional behavior (disruptive behavior). These examples can, in part, be integrated into a code of conduct for acceptable and disruptive (or inappropriate) behaviors.

Creating and Implementing a Process for Managing Disruptive Behavior

Once a code of conduct has been designed and agreed to, it is important to begin the process of designing the process to manage disruptive behavior. The Joint Commission is not specific about how the process itself is delineated, only that it be created and implemented. The organizationwide development of a process to manage disruptive behavior should involve the following principles and/or elements:
- Developing and disseminating a code of conduct
- Reviewing and learning lessons from collected data on previous incidents of disruptive behavior
- Educating staff on acceptable behavior
- Defining disruptive behavior
- Creating processes for managing disruptive behavior
- Maintaining leadership unity on interventions
- Developing leadership skills for managing disruptive behavior
- Fostering a team approach in the organization
- Encouraging individuals to report disruptive behaviors
- Conducting periodic surveys on the climate or culture of the organization

How an organization chooses to construct its process depends on the needs of the organization and how complex the issue has been in the past. In fact, using collected data to consider when designing the process can be particularly informative.

It is also important to have a consistent, team-based approach to designing the process. Ensure that the right people are involved: executive leadership (medical staff, nursing, and so on), risk management, human resources, department heads, the board of directors (or a member), quality improvement/management, legal counsel, midlevel management, representation of all kinds

Sidebar 4-1

Behavioral Descriptors for Modeling Professionalism and/or Describing Violations of Professionalism ("Disruptive" Behaviors)

Professional (Appropriate) Behaviors

- Encourages clear, direct, and honest communication
- Accepts constructive feedback
- Demonstrates respect for staff input into clinical care
- Responds to pages in a timely, civil manner
- Responds to requests in a cooperative manner
- Offers constructive input during patient care decision making
- Cooperates in quality assurance activities
- Arranges and cooperates for coverage when not available
- Demonstrates respect for patients and their family members
- Clarifies points of agreement and disagreement in patient care deliberations
- Accepts feedback in a civil and receptive manner
- Respects patient's need for confidentiality
- Handles staff problems or dilemmas in a cooperative, respectful manner
- Focuses on real, manageable issues
- Chooses appropriate timing to bring up problems for discussion
- Encourages others to express enthusiasm and input
- Offers appreciation and affirmation to peers/coworkers when they function well
- Focuses on accomplishing common interests, goals, and work objectives
- Accepts the inevitability of mistakes as a learning opportunity
- Constructively tries to repair system failures or problems
- Sets aside quality time for relationship building with peers/staff
- Reliably demonstrates patient care in adherence to agreed-upon standards
- Does equitable share of work compared to legitimate sample of peers

Violations of Professionalism

- Threatens retribution or litigation
- Consistently demonstrates threatening behavior (validly witnessed)
- Uses ethnic or gender slurs in threatening or intimidating fashion
- Openly denigrates colleagues in front of staff/patients
- Compulsively tries to win arguments at someone else's expense
- Regularly displays anger or shouting outbursts
- Consistently offers cynical, sarcastic, or caustic remarks
- Sidesteps or violates agreed-upon call and vacation or scheduling policies
- Consistently distracts or brings up old issues when dealing with a current item of discussion
- Regularly shifts blame for implied, intimated, or actual negative outcomes
- Uses degrading, abusive, or sarcastic language at an identifiable target
- Engages in "unwelcome" sexual advances
- Shames peers or staff (or administration) for negative outcomes
- Engages in patient "dumping," or call-dumping
- Criticizes colleagues/staff in inappropriate public forums
- Regularly uses intimidation toward peers, those in lesser-power roles, and others with a direct relationship to specific patient care actions
- Consistently disregards practice rules, standards, or ethical policies

Source: John-Henry Pfifferling, Center for Professional Well-Being, 2006. Reprinted with permission.

📝 For Your Consideration

Take a moment to brainstorm unacceptable or disruptive behaviors you have witnessed or experienced during your tenure in the health care field and note those behaviors in the following worksheet. Also, fill in some acceptable or appropriate behaviors that you have witnessed or considered essential to promoting a healthy work environment.

Acceptable or Appropriate Behaviors (for example, "respect")	Disruptive or Inappropriate Behaviors (for example, "intimidation")

of staff in the organization, and other staff who will have to interact with the process in some way or other. It is also important that various perspectives from different departments and areas of care be represented. This can all happen in one meeting, where people verbalize ideas or concerns, or it can take the form of a private, anonymous survey.

The process should include a few key elements: a definition of disruptive behavior, education for staff on disruptive behavior, examples of unacceptable and acceptable behaviors, and a written process that clearly delineates the steps taken to deal with any incidents of disruptive behavior. The process should include a reporting process, an investigation that takes into consideration the severity of the violation, the presence of any mitigating factors, and any harm done to patients.[2] The process must also define what staff positions must be involved in the process along the way (for example, "The initiating complaint should be submitted to the staff member's direct manager or service chief."). There may be additional committees or individuals already functioning in the organization that can be of great help when dealing with disruptive behavior. These could include any wellness or staff health committees, social workers, staff psychologists or therapists, and so on. It may also be necessary at some point in the process to bring in external professional assistance to help defuse a particularly difficult situation or refer a staff member to an external evaluating agency, though organization leadership should still remain engaged in the process.

An important component of any process is the organization's commitment to following through, no matter how uncomfortable or stressful it may be to deal with. For a staff member who is unwilling to adjust his or her behavior after a verified report of disruptive behavior, an escalation of consequences should be integrated into the policy; this shows that the organization takes its commitment to zero tolerance seriously and helps reassure staff who have been victimized that their voice is heard. The following are examples of the kinds of steps that can and should be taken when implementing a process to manage disruptive behavior:

1. Submit a confidential report of the disruptive behavior to a manager. In the case where the disruptive behavior is being reported by a staff member about his or her manager, there should be additional reporting channels.
2. Notify manager/leader of the staff member who was reported.
3. Investigate report. All parties are informed confidentially, and interviews take place. This process can be facilitated by the human resources department. The defendant must be notified of the complaint and given a chance to respond. The complainant must be made aware that action is being taken. Inherently linked to this step is a clear non-retaliation policy. Staff who file a complaint must feel safe to do so and not be wary of retaliation.
4. Design a solution to correct and defuse disruptive behavior. The disruptive staff member and his or her manager must agree to this solution (the agreement and plan of action are put in writing and signed by the disruptive staff member and his or her manager/chief/leader), and it should include milestones and goals. This plan also includes a "consequence clause," which defines the escalating consequences if compliance with the plan is not achieved. It is important to note that the corrective action should be commensurate with the behavior and any violations of state or federal law should always be taken into consideration (for example, for a disruptive staff member who threatened another staff member with violence, a mandatory enrollment in an anger management course may be part of the corrective action, whereas in the case of a staff member actually assaulting another staff member, legal or criminal action will most likely be involved). *Note: This step may also include the involvement of additional staff such as the physician wellness committee, staff wellness committee, a staff or contracted psychologist, an employee assistance program, and so on.*
5. Monitor the plan and note progress according to the milestones set.
6. If successful completion of the plan is achieved, note and acknowledge it.
7. If the disruptive staff member is unable to comply with the plan of action, enact escalating consequences. This stage may repeat, depending on the nature of the behavior and kind of remedial action under way.
8. If the disruptive staff member is still unwilling to comply with the plan after consequences are put in place and repeated attempts to remediate the behavior have been taken, terminate the staff member, if warranted, based on the decision made by the "deciding body or party."

Designing a Process: Additional Steps to Consider
When designing a process, it can be helpful to allow some degree of anonymity, particularly if it relates to patient safety concerns. For example, a staff member may not feel comfortable reporting a complaint directly about another staff member if he or she is more concerned about a process than about the behavioral habits of one person in particular. In these cases, the staff member should be aware of an anonymous reporting

option, but this should be used more for reporting patient safety concerns or process concerns. Allowing staff to randomly report concerns about staff members in an anonymous way could encourage unnecessary and unfounded complaints about staff for the purposes of "getting them in trouble" rather than reporting a legitimate problem.

Also, in all steps, there is a need for consistency and fairness in the approach. This kind of process should never be manipulated for the sake of eliminating a staff member or to punish one while others remain untouched. For a process to be considered valid and effective, it must be implemented broadly and enforced fairly.

Also integrated into a process like this should be the indication of assisting the staff member who is disruptive to overcome his or her behavior and be assisted to become (or return to being) an effective, supported, and valued member of the team. Being reported and guided through a disruptive behavior process should never be viewed of as a death sentence or a sign that the staff member is expected to leave the organization. The goal of the process should be essentially positive (to help the staff member become a more productive part of the team) and take all the possible steps available (within reason and without causing any additional damage to the work environment) to help the staff member overcome his or her disruptive behavior.

Another important and necessary element to consider in designing a process is to ensure that all those affected by the disruptive behavior are taken into consideration when planning improvements or interventions. Additional staff may need an opportunity to share their concerns, or they may need additional assistance to feel positive about their work environment. The pervasive impact of disruptive behavior can cause an organization to function in a dysfunctional or toxic manner, and this may mean that the staff need training or skills development in such areas as communication, teamwork, and providing constructive feedback. All these steps, if warranted, should be developed and integrated into any planned process to deal with the disruptive behavior.

Most important is the need to apply a flexible and responsive approach to any designed process. As staffing needs and styles change, so should the processes in place to deal with staff and organizational issues. For example, if an organization changes the kinds of care, treatment, and services it provides and, as a result, begins to work with new staff or new types of staff, the

processes in place should be adapted to accommodate those changes. This is particularly important when it relates to difficult situations, such as disruptive behavior. Any inconsistency in approach can have a demoralizing impact on staff in general and actually serve to perpetuate the negative impact of disruptive behavior.

Accommodating the Different Staffing Types in the Organization

When designing a process for dealing with disruptive behavior, it is important to take into consideration the various types of staff members that interact with the organization. This helps ensure that the process is applied in a universal manner while accommodating (or speaking to) the different types of structures under which those staff members are managed or monitored.

In some types of health care organizations, the health care workers that provide services for the organization can have different kinds of interactive relationships with the organization. For example, some are full-time employees, some are contracted staff, others are temporary staff, and yet others are affiliated with the organization through the medical staff bylaws only. The issue of different types of staff and the various ways they are managed should be taken into consideration when designing the process for the organization. In the "For Your Consideration" chart on page 57, take a moment to inventory the different ways that staff operate at your health care organization and what policies or procedures you may (or may not) have in place to deal with them. It is important to note that while some of these positions (such as medical staff) do not exist at all types of health care organizations, there may be times when your organization has to interact with them, so it can be helpful to consider whether you have a process or policy in place for that relationship or whether you even can or need to. In cases in which you do not have a formal, contractual relationship with a staff member who interacts with your organization but who is disruptive, it can be helpful to determine the options you do have to report a concern.

Della Lin, M.D., executive director, CME, at The Queens Medical Center in Honolulu, Hawaii, suggests considering the following reccomendations in designing a code of conduct and a process to deal with disruptive behavior:

- Ensure that everyone is on the same page. Involve all relevant staff, including legal counsel, leadership, and the board of directors, for example. Ensure that the code takes into consideration any unique issues that could affect the organization and how the code should be delineated or thought

For Your Consideration

	Type of Staff	Policies and Procedures in Place for Disciplinary Action/Staffing Policies	Comment
Category 1	Full-time staff of the organization, including physicians		
Category 2	Contracted staff		
Category 3	Employees of physicians with privileges		
Category 4	Physicians with privileges		
Additional Categories			

out. For example, "We're a small rural hospital, and we have a disruptive physician who is our only obstetrician," or "Our nurses are unionized."

- Be clear. Ensure that the policy and code are clearly delineated and disseminated among all staff. Remind everyone that zero tolerance is the goal. This helps prevent instances of "No one told me about *this* before."
- Articulate the process clearly. Ensure that the intervention process is clearly explained and clarified with all staff. There is often a multistep process involved, with the first step being staff signing an agreement to abide by the code of conduct and that they are aware of the multistep process to deal with disruptive behavior.
- Delineate how anyone in the organization can bring disruptive behavior concerns to leadership and make sure it is understood that the issue will not "die" there. Ensure that you have a system in place for follow-up and action. Avoid letting staff feel like their reported concerns have dropped into a black hole.
- Always consider patient safety and patient care first. Poor behavior is really not much different from incompetence, Lin points out, as they both affect the ability of others to get their jobs done.[1]

In their article on disruptive clinician behavior, Grena Porto, R.N., M.S., A.R.M., C.P.H.R.M., and Richard Lauve, M.D., M.B.A., C.P.E., F.A.C.P.E., outline a series of principles for organizations to keep in mind when approaching this issue, including the following points:

- Universal code of conduct
- Planned implementation of a universal code of conduct
- Compliance monitoring
- Non-retaliation provisions. Compliance monitoring must be complemented by a clear policy of non-retaliation.
- Code enforcement. In order for an organization to effectively reduce or eliminate the incidence of disruptive behavior, it must reinforce the policy consistently and with all staff in the organization. No one should be exempt from the policy.
- Flexibility. The organization must offer all available resources for coaching and mentoring staff when necessary. The goal is to correct the behavior, not eliminate the individual.
- Oversight committee. A multidisciplinary committee must be appointed to monitor the implementation of the code as well as violations to that code.

- Preventive strategies. There should be additional strategies in place to help prevent disruptive behavior. This can include building stronger relationships among staff, teamwork training, and training in communication with standardized communication techniques such as Situation–Background–Assessment–Recommendation (SBAR).[2]

The following examples of processes and policies are currently in use in health care organizations around the country. While many of them relate specifically to either medical staff or a hospital setting (and that may not apply to your type of health care organization), the principles provide important guidance and structure to how processes can be designed and implemented.

Figure 4-1 provides an example of a medical code of professional behavior being used at a hospital. While not all types of health care organizations have medical staff, this figure provides some helpful examples of types of elements that could be integrated into a code of conduct.

Figure 4-2, pages 65–67, provides an example of a disruptive behavior policy. This policy covers dealing with both staff (medical staff in this instance) and students.

Figure 4-3, page 68, provides another example of an organization's policy and code of conduct relating to disruptive behavior and medical staff. While not all organizations may have a medical staff, the principles included therein provide helpful examples to consider while drafting a policy and code of conduct.

The Health or Wellness Committee

Establishing or working with an existing health committee can be helpful in designing a process to deal with disruptive behavior. "We are seeing a common trend now where organizations are adding the issue of disruptive behavior to their work on substance or alcohol abuse or other impairment issues," notes Bill Swiggart, M.A., training director at the Center for Professional Health (CPH) at Vanderbilt. In recent years, Swiggart notes, Vanderbilt has begun offering a course for distressed physicians at CPH in addition to courses on sexual boundaries and substance abuse.

Figure 4-1. Stanford Hospital & Clinics and Lucile Packard Children's Hospital Medical Staff Code of Professional Behavior

This policy applies to: ☑ ***Stanford Hospital and Clinics*** ☑ ***Lucile Packard Children's Hospital***	**Date Written or Last Revision:** *Written 1997* *Revised: May 2006*
Name of Policy: Disruptive Behavior of Medical Staff and Physicians-in-Training Policy	**Page 1 of 6**
Departments Affected: All Departments	

I. **PURPOSE**

To ensure Medical Staff members and Physicians-in-Training (Practitioners) conduct themselves in a professional, cooperative and appropriate manner while providing services as a Practitioner at SHC or LPCH.

To encourage the prompt identification and resolution of alleged disruptive behavior by all involved or affected persons through informal, collaborative efforts at counseling and rehabilitation that are intended to achieve any required behavior modification by the Practitioner.

To provide a formal procedure for the further investigation and resolution of disruptive behavior by Practitioners which has not been appropriately modified by prior informal efforts.

To provide for the appropriate discipline of Practitioners only after the informal efforts and formal procedures described in this Policy have been unsuccessful in causing the Practitioner to appropriately modify behavior in compliance with this Policy.

II. **DEFINITIONS**

A. Practitioner
1. Any member of the Medical Staff of SHC or LPCH (which includes physicians, dentists, podiatrists, psychologists) and any intern, resident, or fellow at either facility.

III. **POLICY STATEMENT**

It is the policy of the Medical Staff of SHC and LPCH that all Practitioners who are members of, or affiliated with, the Medical Staff or with any physician training program at these facilities (i.e. residency, fellowship) shall conduct themselves in a professional and cooperative manner, and shall not engage in disruptive behavior.

(continued)

Figure 4-1. Stanford Hospital & Clinics and Lucile Packard Children's Hospital Medical Staff Code of Professional Behavior, *continued*

This policy applies to: ☑ ***Stanford Hospital and Clinics*** ☑ ***Lucile Packard Children's Hospital***	**Date Written or Last Revision:** *Written 1997* *Revised: May 2006*
Name of Policy: Disruptive Behavior of Medical Staff and Physicians-in-Training Policy	**Page 2 of 6**
Departments Affected: All Departments	

Disruptive behavior includes, but is not limited to:
-- conduct that interferes with the provision of quality patient care
-- conduct that constitutes sexual harassment
-- making or threatening reprisals for reporting disruptive behavior
-- shouting or using vulgar or profane or abusive language
-- abusive behavior towards patients or staff
-- physical assault
-- intimidating behavior
-- refusal to cooperate with other staff members

IV.   **PROCEDURES**

A.   The Medical Staff encourages collegial and educational efforts by leaders and management to address questions relating to an individual's clinical practice and/or professional conduct. The goal of these efforts is to arrive at voluntary, responsive actions by the individual to resolve the questions that have been raised. Collegial efforts may include, but are not limited to, counseling, sharing of comparative data, monitoring, focused review, and additional training or education.

The relevant medical staff leader shall determine whether it is appropriate to include documentation of collegial intervention efforts in an individual's confidential file. If documentation is included in an individual's file, the individual will have an opportunity to review it and respond in writing. The response shall be maintained in the individual's file along with the original documentation.

Collegial intervention efforts are encouraged, but are not mandatory, and shall be within the discretion of the appropriate medical staff leaders.

B.   Although the Medical Staff encourages the persons directly involved to informally resolve incidents of disruptive behavior by a Practitioner, it is recognized that, for various reasons, such a resolution may be impracticable. Therefore, any written or oral report of alleged disruptive Practitioner behavior may be sent to the Chief of Staff, who shall initiate an informal investigation as he/she deems appropriate to identify or rule out the existence of disruptive behavior.

(continued)

Figure 4-1. Stanford Hospital & Clinics and Lucile Packard Children's Hospital Medical Staff Code of Professional Behavior, *continued*

This policy applies to: ☑ *Stanford Hospital and Clinics* ☑ *Lucile Packard Children's Hospital*	**Date Written or Last Revision:** *Written 1997* *Revised: May 2006*
Name of Policy: Disruptive Behavior of Medical Staff and Physicians-in-Training Policy	**Page 3 of 6**
Departments Affected: All Departments	

C. At some point during this investigation, the Chief of Staff will meet with the Practitioner to review the alleged behavior and the requirements of this Policy. Both the Chief of Staff and the Practitioner may be accompanied at this meeting by such other practitioners as the Chief of Staff or the Practitioner feel are necessary to explain the alleged disruptive behavior. At the completion of such investigation, the Chief of Staff will make a determination as to whether the Practitioner engaged in disruptive behavior.

   1. If the Chief of Staff determines that the Practitioner has not engaged in disruptive behavior, he/she will advise the Practitioner and the person to whom the allegedly disruptive behavior was directed of such determination, and will prepare a written report of such determination to be filed in the Chief of Staff's file, with a copy to be given to the Practitioner.

   2. If the Chief of Staff determines that the Practitioner has engaged in disruptive behavior, he/she will meet with the Practitioner to counsel the Practitioner concerning compliance with this Policy and assist the Practitioner in identifying methods for structuring professional and working relationships and resolving problems without disruptive behavior. It is the intent of this Policy to allow the Chief of Staff latitude to develop any plan for resolution that is deemed appropriate with the goal to achieve a modification of the Practitioner's behavior. The Chief of Staff will also perform the functions described in Paragraphs 3, 4, and 5 of this Policy.

D. Following the meeting(s) with the Practitioner, the Chief of Staff may, at his or her discretion, arrange for and participate in a meeting between the Practitioner and the person(s) toward whom the disruptive behavior was directed. In determining whether to arrange such a meeting, the Chief of Staff is to consider the wishes of the person(s) who reported the disruptive behavior. If no such meeting is arranged, the Chief of Staff will meet with the person(s) toward whom the disruptive behavior was directed, to advise of the resolution of the matter.

(continued)

Figure 4-1. Stanford Hospital & Clinics and Lucile Packard Children's Hospital Medical Staff Code of Professional Behavior, *continued*

This policy applies to: ☑ ***Stanford Hospital and Clinics*** ☑ ***Lucile Packard Children's Hospital***	**Date Written or Last Revision:** *Written 1997* *Revised: May 2006*
Name of Policy: Disruptive Behavior of Medical Staff and Physicians-in-Training Policy	**Page 4 of 6**
Departments Affected: All Departments	

E. Following the meeting(s) with the Practitioner, and the person(s) toward whom the disruptive behavior was directed as applicable, the Chief of Staff will prepare a written summary of the reported behavior and the meetings to document the first violation of this Policy. In preparing the written summary of the reported behavior, the Chief of Staff should document all of the following: a) the date and time of the questionable behavior, b) if the behavior affected or involved a patient and if so the patient's name and medical record number, c) the circumstances that precipitated the behavior, d) a factual, objective description of the behavior, e) the consequences of the behavior for patient care or hospital operations, f) the dates, times and participants in any meetings with the Practitioner, staff, etc. about the behavior. The summary will be filed in the Chief of Staff's file, the Practitioner's credentials file, and a copy will be given to the Practitioner. The Chief of Staff will also inform the Practitioner's Chief of Service of this violation.

F. The Chief of Staff will also develop a plan for monitoring future compliance with or violation of this Policy, and will document findings of these reviews in writing to the Practitioner's credentials file and the Chief of Staff's file, with copies to the Practitioner.

G. If a second report of alleged disruptive behavior is made concerning the same Practitioner, the Chief of Staff will prepare a memo referring the matter to the Well Being of Physicians and Physicians-in-Training Committee. The Practitioner's Chief of Service will be copied on this memo. The Committee will meet with the Practitioner and attempt to further assist the Practitioner in identifying methods for structuring professional and working relationships and resolving problems without disruptive behavior. Referrals for counseling with required reports to the Committee may also be a part of this process. It is the intent of this Policy to allow the Committee latitude to develop any plan for resolution that is deemed appropriate with the goal of rehabilitating the Practitioner. This Committee will also develop a plan for monitoring future compliance with or violation of this Policy. At its discretion, the Committee may consult with those person(s) who were the object(s) of the disruptive behavior. Finally, this Committee will send a written report to the Chief of Staff when the Committee has concluded its work with the Practitioner.

H. The Committee report shall remain in the Chief of Staff's file of the Practitioner, and the Practitioner's credentials file.

(continued)

Figure 4-1. Stanford Hospital & Clinics and Lucile Packard Children's Hospital Medical Staff Code of Professional Behavior, *continued*

This policy applies to: ☑ ***Stanford Hospital and Clinics*** ☑ ***Lucile Packard Children's Hospital***	**Date Written or Last Revision:** *Written 1997* *Revised: May 2006*
Name of Policy: Disruptive Behavior of Medical Staff and Physicians-in-Training Policy	**Page 5 of 6**
Departments Affected: All Departments	

    I.   Failure of the Committee to satisfactorily resolve the behavior problem will result in a referral of the matter for further review and possible discipline as outlined in the Medical Staff Bylaws.

V.   RELATED DOCUMENTS

    A.   Joint Commission on Accreditation of Healthcare Organizations Manual
    B.   Well Being Committee Brochure

VI.   APPENDICES

    A.   None

VII.   DOCUMENT INFORMATION

    A.   Legal Authority/References
        1.   Hospital legal counsel

    B.   Author/Original Date
        Lawrence Shuer, M.D., SHC Chief of Staff
        SHC/LPCH Well Being Committee
        1997

    C.   Gatekeeper of Original Document
        Medical Staff Services

    D.   Distribution and Training Requirements
        1.   This policy resides in the Administrative Manuals of both hospitals.
        2.   New documents or any revised documents will be distributed to Administrative Manual holders. This policy is on the Medical Staff Services website and is distributed to all Medical Staff at time of initial appointment

    E.   Review and Renewal Requirements
        This policy will be reviewed and/or revised every three years or as required by change of law or practice.

    F.   Review and Revision History

(continued)

Figure 4-1. Stanford Hospital & Clinics and Lucile Packard Children's Hospital Medical Staff Code of Professional Behavior, *continued*

This policy applies to: ☑ **Stanford Hospital and Clinics** ☑ **Lucile Packard Children's Hospital**	**Date Written or Last Revision:** *Written 1997* *Revised: May 2006*
Name of Policy: Disruptive Behavior of Medical Staff and Physicians-in-Training Policy	**Page 6 of 6**
Departments Affected: All Departments	

Written 1997
Reviewed 2000
Reviewed and revised 2003; 2006

G.   Approvals
    Well Being Committee   Jan, 2003
    SHC Medical Board   Feb, 2003; July 2006
    LPCH Medical Board   Feb, 2003; July 2006
    SHC Board of Directors   Feb, 2003; July 2006
    LPCH Board of Directors   Feb, 2003; July 2006

This document is intended for use by staff of Stanford Hospital & Clinics and/or Lucile Packard Children's Hospital.
No representations or warranties are made for outside use.
Not for outside reproduction or publication without permission.

Source: Stanford Hospital & Clinics, Stanford, CA. Reprinted with permission.

In the following excerpt from Temple University Hospital's Web site, the Physicians' Health Committee provides background on why the committee was formed, what its purpose is, and how the process works.

Why Was the Physicians' Health Committee (PHC) Formed?

The practice of medicine is a demanding profession. We are committed to ensuring the health and well-being of our physicians and their families so they can continue to provide the finest care and teaching to our patients and students.

We recognize that any physical, mental, and emotional problems that affect our physicians' performance also affect their patients, colleagues, and families. We understand that, although such problems are usually treatable, they often may be ignored or left untreated.

We believe that treatment and/or rehabilitation is the best way to address any such problem.

What Does the Committee Do?

The PHC is responsible for reaching out to physicians on staff at Temple University Hospital whose performance has become impaired by physical, mental, or emotional problems or by substance abuse.

We are advocates for those physicians and their families, colleagues, and patients. We take or recommend actions or treatments that are in the best interests of the impaired physicians and the community they serve.

(continued on page 69)

Figure 4-2. Stanford Hospital & Clinics and Lucile Packard Children's Hospital Disruptive Behavior of Medical Staff and Physicians-in-Training Policy

This policy applies to:
 Stanford Hospital & Clinics (SHC)
 Lucile Packard Children's Hospital (LPCH)

Date Written or Last Revision:
Written 1997
Revised: May 2006
Name of Policy:
Disruptive Behavior of Medical Staff and Physicians-in-Training Policy
Departments Affected:
All Departments

I. PURPOSE

To ensure Medical Staff members and Physicians-in-Training (Practitioners) conduct themselves in a professional, cooperative and appropriate manner while providing services as a Practitioner at SHC or LPCH.

To encourage the prompt identification and resolution of alleged disruptive behavior by all involved or affected persons through informal, collaborative efforts at counseling and rehabilitation that are intended to achieve any required behavior modification by the Practitioner.

To provide a formal procedure for the further investigation and resolution of disruptive behavior by Practitioners which has not been appropriately modified by prior informal efforts.

To provide for the appropriate discipline of Practitioners only after the informal efforts and formal procedures described in this Policy have been unsuccessful in causing the Practitioner to appropriately modify behavior in compliance with this Policy.

II. DEFINITIONS
 A. Practitioner
  1. Any member of the Medical Staff of SHC or LPCH (which includes physicians, dentists, podiatrists, psychologists) and any intern, resident, or fellow at either facility.

III. POLICY STATEMENT
 It is the policy of the Medical Staff of SHC and LPCH that all Practitioners who are members of, or affiliated with, the Medical Staff or with any physician training program at these facilities (i.e., residency, fellowship) shall conduct themselves in a professional and cooperative manner, and shall not engage in disruptive behavior.

 Disruptive behavior includes, but is not limited to:
 –conduct that interferes with the provision of quality patient care
 –conduct that constitutes sexual harassment
 –making or threatening reprisals for reporting disruptive behavior
 –shouting or using vulgar or profane or abusive language
 –abusive behavior towards patients or staff
 –physical assault
 –intimidating behavior
 –refusal to cooperate with other staff members

IV. PROCEDURES
 A. The Medical Staff encourages collegial and educational efforts by leaders and management to address questions relating to an individual's clinical practice and/or professional conduct. The goal of these efforts is to arrive at voluntary, responsive actions by the individual to resolve the questions that have been raised. Collegial efforts may include, but are not limited to, counseling, sharing of comparative data, monitoring, focused review, and additional training or education.

(continued)

Figure 4-2. Stanford Hospital & Clinics and Lucile Packard Children's Hospital Disruptive Behavior of Medical Staff and Physicians-in-Training Policy, *continued*

The relevant medical staff leader shall determine whether it is appropriate to include documentation of collegial intervention efforts in an individual's confidential file. If documentation is included in an individual's file, the individual will have an opportunity to review it and respond in writing.

The response shall be maintained in the individual's file along with the original documentation. Collegial intervention efforts are encouraged, but are not mandatory, and shall be within the discretion of the appropriate medical staff leaders.

B. Although the Medical Staff encourages the persons directly involved to informally resolve incidents of disruptive behavior by a Practitioner, it is recognized that, for various reasons, such a resolution may be impracticable. Therefore, any written or oral report of alleged disruptive Practitioner behavior may be sent to the Chief of Staff, who shall initiate an informal investigation as he/she deems appropriate to identify or rule out the existence of disruptive behavior.

C. At some point during this investigation, the Chief of Staff will meet with the Practitioner to review the alleged behavior and the requirements of this Policy. Both the Chief of Staff and the Practitioner may be accompanied at this meeting by such other practitioners as the Chief of Staff or the Practitioner feel are necessary to explain the alleged disruptive behavior. At the completion of such investigation, the Chief of Staff will make a determination as to whether the Practitioner engaged in disruptive behavior.
   1. If the Chief of Staff determines that the Practitioner has not engaged in disruptive behavior, he/she will advise the Practitioner and the person to whom the allegedly disruptive behavior was directed of such determination, and will prepare a written report of such determination to be filed in the Chief of Staff's file, with a copy to be given to the Practitioner.
   2. If the Chief of Staff determines that the Practitioner has engaged in disruptive behavior, he/she will meet with the Practitioner to counsel the Practitioner concerning compliance with this Policy and assist the Practitioner in identifying methods for structuring professional and working relationships and resolving problems without disruptive behavior. It is the intent of this Policy to allow the Chief of Staff latitude to develop any plan for resolution that is deemed appropriate with the goal to achieve a modification of the Practitioner's behavior. The Chief of Staff will also perform the functions described in Paragraphs 3, 4, and 5 of this Policy.

D. Following the meeting(s) with the Practitioner, the Chief of Staff may, at his or her discretion, arrange for and participate in a meeting between the Practitioner and the person(s) toward whom the disruptive behavior was directed. In determining whether to arrange such a meeting, the Chief of Staff is to consider the wishes of the person(s) who reported the disruptive behavior. If no such meeting is arranged, the Chief of Staff will meet with the person(s) toward whom the disruptive behavior was directed, to advise of the resolution of the matter.

E. Following the meeting(s) with the Practitioner, and the person(s) toward whom the disruptive behavior was directed as applicable, the Chief of Staff will prepare a written summary of the reported behavior and the meetings to document the first violation of this Policy. In preparing the written summary of the reported behavior, the Chief of Staff should document all of the following: a) the date and time of the questionable behavior, b) if the behavior affected or involved a patient and if so the patient's name and medical record number, c) the circumstances that precipitated the behavior, d) a factual, objective description of the behavior, e) the consequences of the behavior for patient care or hospital operations, f) the dates, times and participants in any meetings with the Practitioner, staff, etc. about the behavior. The summary will be filed in the Chief of Staff's file, the Practitioner's credentials file, and a copy will be given to the Practitioner. The Chief of Staff will also inform the Practitioner's Chief of Service of this violation.

F. The Chief of Staff will also develop a plan for monitoring future compliance with or violation of this Policy, and will document findings of these reviews in writing to the Practitioner's credentials file and the Chief of Staff's file, with copies to the Practitioner.

G. If a second report of alleged disruptive behavior is made concerning the same Practitioner, the Chief of Staff will prepare a memo referring the matter to the Well Being of Physicians and Physicians-in-Training Committee. The Practitioner's Chief of Service will be copied on this memo. The Committee will meet with the Practitioner and attempt to further assist the Practitioner in identifying methods for structuring professional and working relationships and resolving problems without disruptive behavior. Referrals for counseling with required reports to the Committee may also be a part of this process. It is the intent of this Policy to allow the Committee latitude to develop any plan for resolution that is deemed appropriate with the goal of rehabilitating the Practitioner. This Committee will also develop a plan for monitoring future compliance with or violation of this Policy. At its discretion, the Committee may consult with those person(s) who were the object(s) of the disruptive behavior. Finally, this Committee will send a written report to the Chief of Staff when the Committee has concluded its work with the Practitioner.

(continued)

Figure 4-2. Stanford Hospital & Clinics and Lucile Packard Children's Hospital Disruptive Behavior of Medical Staff and Physicians-in-Training Policy, *continued*

H. The Committee report shall remain in the Chief of Staff's file of the Practitioner, and the Practitioner's credentials file.

I. Failure of the Committee to satisfactorily resolve the behavior problem will result in a referral of the matter for further review and possible discipline as outlined in the Medical Staff Bylaws.

V. RELATED DOCUMENTS
A. Joint Commission on Accreditation of Healthcare Organizations Manual

B. Well Being Committee Brochure

VI. APPENDICES
A. None

VII. DOCUMENT INFORMATION
A. Legal Authority/References
   1. Hospital legal counsel

B. Author/Original Date
   Lawrence Shuer, M.D., SHC Chief of Staff
   SHC/LPCH Well Being Committee
   1997

C. Gatekeeper of Original Document
   Medical Staff Services

D. Distribution and Training Requirements
   1. This policy resides in the Administrative Manuals of both hospitals.
   2. New documents or any revised documents will be distributed to Administrative Manual holders. This policy is on the Medical Staff Services website and is distributed to all Medical Staff at time of initial appointment

E. Review and Renewal Requirements
   This policy will be reviewed and/or revised every three years or as required by change of law or practice.

F. Review and Revision History
   Written 1997
   Reviewed 2000
   Reviewed and revised 2003; 2006

G. Approvals
   Well Being Committee Jan, 2003
   SHC Medical Board Feb, 2003; July 2006
   LPCH Medical Board Feb, 2003; July 2006
   SHC Board of Directors Feb, 2003; July 2006
   LPCH Board of Directors Feb, 2003; July 2006

Source: Lawrence Shuer, Stanford Hospital & Clinics, Stanford, CA. Reprinted with permission.

Figure 4-3. HealthPartners—Regions Hospital: Medical Staff Code of Conduct Policies—Disruptive Medical Staff

The purpose of this policy is to ensure optimum patient care by promoting a safe, cooperative and professional health care environment and to prevent or eliminate conduct which disrupts the operation of the Hospital, adversely affects the ability of others to do their jobs, creates a hostile work environment for Hospital employees or other Medical Staff members, or interferes with an individual's ability to practice competently.

This policy applies to all Regions Hospital Medical Staff members and Allied Health Professional Staff.

Unacceptable and disruptive conduct may include, but is not limited to, behavior such as:
* Verbal attacks or verbal abuse directed at other appointees to the Medical Staff, and Hospital personnel including nursing staff or patients. Verbal attacks may be judged on content, tone and level of voice.
* Impertinent and inappropriate comments or illustrations made in patient medical records or other official documents.
* Non-constructive criticism addressed to its recipient in such a way as to intimidate, undermine confidence or imply stupidity or incompetence.
* Physically abusive behavior leveled at other appointees to the Medical Staff, Hospital personnel including nursing staff or patients. Physical abuse is subject to the Regions Hospital workplace violence policy.

It is the official policy of Regions Hospital that all individuals within its facilities be treated courteously, respectfully and with dignity. To that end, Regions Hospital requires Medical Staff members and Allied Health Professional staff members to conduct themselves in a professional and cooperative manner while present on the Regions Hospital campus. If a Regions Hospital Staff member or Allied Health Professional Staff member fails to conduct him or herself in this manner, the matter shall be addressed in accordance with this policy. It is the intention of Regions Hospital that this policy is enforced in a fair and equitable manner while maintaining the welfare, safety and security of all involved.

Procedure:
1. A single <u>substantiated</u> egregious incident, including but not limited to assault, felony convictions, fraudulent acts, stealing, throwing equipment/records, or inappropriate physical behavior may result in summary suspension, pending investigation by the Chief of Staff, Vice President of Medical Affairs, or the Chief Executive Officer of the Hospital.
2. If the incident does not require summary suspension, the procedure outlined on the flow diagram will be followed. In summary, the incident will be appropriately investigated and documented by interviewing the individuals involved and the individual accused. The Chief of Staff (or designee) will coordinate the investigation. An attempt will be made to identify underlying problems which contributed to the incident and which may require some type of intervention. If this is the first substantiated incident reported, Warning #1 will be issued. The appropriate feedback to those involved in the incident will be made. The Chief of Staff (or designee) will arrange for appropriate follow-up with the individual accused.
3. For second and third substantiated incidents reported, the process will be followed as outlined in the flow diagram. A second substantiated incident will warrant the issuance of Warning #2, which will require appropriate evaluation and behavioral intervention.
4. A third substantiated incident will require review by the Medical Executive Committee, which may result in a recommendation to the Governing Board for removal of the individual from the medical staff and loss of all privileges at Regions Hospital.
   a. Incident #1/Warning #1: This behavior is not acceptable and it must not occur again; apologies to staff involved are required. A report in the form of a letter is sent to the credentialing file and the Division/Section Head.
   b. Incident #2/Warning #2: The same as Warning #1. After a second warning, an individual will be required to seek some type of evaluation, counseling and/or behavioral intervention.
   c. Incident #3: Necessitates action by the Medical Executive Committee.
      i. If the incident(s) involve sexual harassment, the Regions Hospital policy regarding sexual harassment by Medical Staff will be followed.
      ii. Prior to any formal action by the Governing Board on the recommendation of the Medical Executive Committee, the Medical Staff member or Allied Health Professional Staff member shall be given formal notice to his/her right to request a hearing pursuant to the Medical Staff Bylaws.
5. In the case of disruptive behavior by a resident or fellow, the director of the training program will meet with the Chief of Staff and/or the Vice President of Medical Affairs. A plan of action will be developed and implemented appropriate to the situation in accordance with the teaching program's policies. In the event that the program is unable or unwilling to deal with the problem, the Regions Hospital policy regarding disruptive Medical Staff will be initiated by the Vice President of Medical Affairs.

Source: Regions Hospital, St. Paul, MN. Used with permission.

We encourage all physicians whose professional performance has been affected and colleagues who become aware of performance issues, to seek help from the committee so that the impaired physician can receive assistance, including early intervention and ease of access to diagnosis, treatment, and rehabilitation.

We assist impaired physicians with enrollment in the Physicians' Health Program of the Pennsylvania Medical Society (PMS).

We protect the privacy of impaired physicians. The identification and treatment process is conducted with strict confidentiality, great discretion, and the highest respect for the individual. We notify only those who have responsibility for the impaired physician's clinical performance.

Equally important, we develop and conduct ongoing programs to educate our staff about physical, mental, and emotional wellness. Our programs focus on teaching physicians and their families about the pressures and conditions that affect physicians in their practice of medicine. We are responsible for increasing awareness about physician wellness, for changing negative attitudes about physician impairment, and for providing factual information about available treatment and rehabilitation programs.

How Does the Referral Process Work?

The services of the committee may be requested through:

Self-referral: A Temple University Hospital physician seeking assistance can call the unstaffed voice mail number (2-COPE / 215-707-2673) to leave a message for the committee. A member of the committee will contact him or her about the nature of the concern and willingness to commit to the appropriate treatment or rehabilitation.

Involuntary referral: The committee will accept referral from any responsible party via the 2-COPE number or through personal contact. The person making the referral will be asked to give his or her name and state the concern. The referring individual's name will not be revealed outside the committee without his or her knowledge or consent.

What Happens After That?

Within three days of the notification, a committee member will be designated to obtain as much firsthand information as possible to evaluate the complaint or concern. Two or more members of the committee will discuss the allegation and, if it appears to be credible, the following actions will be taken as quickly as possible:

The committee member will speak to the physician in question to recommend enrollment in the Physicians' Health Program of the PMS.

The committee member will facilitate referral of the impaired physician to the PMS's Physicians' Health Program for treatment and/or rehabilitation. The committee is responsible for monitoring the effectiveness of the impaired physician's treatment plan in cooperation with the PMS.

The committee member will act as advisor to the appropriate department chairperson and the impaired physician.

When a physician is considered rehabilitated and restored to medical practice, the committee's intervention and responsibility is ended.[3]

Source: Temple University Hospital, Philadelphia, PA. http://www.temple.edu/tuhphc (accessed Aug. 15, 2007)

For Your Consideration

1. Consider the following quote in relation to your organization. What do you think matters most to your staff? Why?

Managers assume that job security is of paramount importance to employees. Among workers, however, it ranks far below desire for respect, a higher standard of management ethics, increased recognition of employee contributions, and closer, more honest communications between employees and senior management.

–Robert H. Rosen

Preventive Medicine for Disruptive Behavior: Fostering a Culture of Safety

One of the most effective ways to prevent disruptive behavior is to create a work environment and work culture that has no room for such negative behavior. A culture of safety in health care, one that promotes safety and a healthy work environment, is an excellent means by which to establish habits and behaviors that can be an effective antidote to disruptive behavior.

In the following example, the imperative for establishing a culture of safety becomes pressing when the environment becomes disruptive in nature due to systemwide changes and poor communication:

The large health system in a bustling West coast city was growing. It boasted two successful, highly rated hospitals, a large network of ambulatory care specialties, a home care and hospice agency, and a skilled nursing home. Now it was growing. The system had recently merged with a smaller system that consisted of a suburban hospital and a smaller network of ambulatory clinics. To streamline its processes and ensure that it was providing consistent, high-quality care to its patients, the new system opted to integrate the clinics that offered similar care, as much as it was reasonable to do so. This meant that some groups came together under one name.

This was not without its challenges. Differing work styles and procedures meant a rocky beginning for some of these groups. Some physicians who had worked well together before the decision to merge were now finding it challenging to work together. A new organizational structure—about which they felt they had little say or knowledge—proved confusing, frustrating, and stressful for the clinic staff. System leadership had communicated the changes and oriented clinic management, but the work environment still did not seem settled. While their commitment to providing high-quality, safe patient care was unquestioned, the steps they were now following seemed discordant and inconsistent. These changes began to take their toll. Tension and territoriality began to emerge among staff, and resentment began to erupt over issues that may not have bothered the staff before the merge—including break times and schedules.

While this scenario does not point to a specific event of disruptive behavior perpetuated by one staff member in particular, the experience of change and rearrangement proved disruptive enough to the staff involved that they began to experience the negative impact of a toxic work environment. The system's leadership was now faced with a growing series of problems in the clinic, which would increase the risk to patient safety and cause other unwelcome effects, such as staff turnover. One effective strategy to help the clinic overcome these challenges and help it find a way to work together is to put in place elements to establish a culture of safety. In a culture of safety, staff members learn important skills and abilities that help them foster a positive work environment that is focused on safe care; this also helps staff develop tools and techniques to work together more cohesively. The following section provides some suggestions to consider in fostering a culture of safety.

Key Skills and Training for Staff to Foster a Culture of Safety

In order for some staff to move beyond a working environment where being disruptive has been the norm and effective communication and teamwork have taken a backseat to steep hierarchies and poor communication, they will need to be empowered and trained on the new skill set that is necessary for a culture of safety to be firmly established. Two important parts of that culture are teamwork and effective communication. While myriad publications and training materials provide a wealth of knowledge and information on these two topics, some of the essential points are highlighted next, particularly as they relate to managing disruptive behavior.

It can be helpful to work closely with the quality improvement/performance improvement staff of your organization to determine which training strategy will be most effective in helping staff master such skills as effective communication and teamwork. It is important to keep in mind, however, that with the perpetrators of disruptive behavior, it can be helpful to reinforce education and training by offering coursework over a period of time rather than offering training in a one-time workshop session. This may be a more effective way of ensuring that the disruptive staff member is more successful at internalizing the messages inherent in the training programs. Additional training can also be integrated into the disruptive staff member's "plan of action."

Teamwork

Clearly, having a process in place to develop and enhance teamwork skills is of great value to a health care organization that is working toward establishing a culture of safety.

While employing a process to deal with disruptive behavior can be helpful and beneficial in ensuring that the roles and responsibilities of the whole health care team are respected, valued, and heard, it is also essential to develop those skills to help staff work as a team. Regardless of the methodology used, some key elements should be in place when developing teamwork:

- Eliminate the hierarchy and focus on collaboration. This does not mean everyone has the same role, but it does mean that everyone has the same opportunity for input and is respected for his or her contribution.
- Specific roles on the team are delineated, respected, and appreciated.
- There is zero tolerance for disruptive behavior, and this mind-set is enforced.
- Team training is made available.

Unfortunately, team training is not usually made available to health care workers while they are in school for their specific skills training, so often a health care organization will have to provide team training to staff once they are in the organization.

"It would be nice to see more staff working together earlier in their careers, like when they are in medical school, pharmacy school, or nursing school," observes Michael Cohen, Pharm.D., president of the Institute for Safe Medication Practices. "It would help forge better working relationships with the different areas of the health care team earlier on and help prevent some of the miscommunications and disruptive behavior that can take place."

The following example of crew resource management can be considered as one of several methodologies that can be applied to help develop teamwork skills and prevent adverse outcomes.

Crew Resource Management as a Teamwork Technique

When the aviation industry began to study the root causes of plane crashes in the late 1970s, it found that approximately half of the crashes were due to human error.[4] Those errors were often linked to the way the team structure in the cockpit—the flight crew—functioned. The original hierarchical structure of the team meant that the captain's word was paramount, and junior staff, despite their concerns about a safety issue or their own wealth of experience and perspective, would rarely question the captain. This led to a number of devastating accidents that cost hundreds of lives.

Subsequently, aviation safety experts began to propose revising the approach to teamwork in the cockpit with a new methodol-

ogy named crew resource management (CRM). Today, this training technique is being used widely by major airlines and military aviation worldwide. In fact, this training is now mandatory for commercial pilots under most regulatory aviation bodies.[4]

CRM training encompasses a wide range of knowledge, skills, and attitudes, including communications, situational awareness, problem solving, decision making, and teamwork, in addition to all the attendant subdisciplines that each of these areas entails. CRM can be defined as a management system that makes optimum use of all available resources—equipment, procedures, and people—to promote safety and enhance the efficiency of flight operations.

There are correlations between aviation and health care: Both have skill-specific positions and high-risk implications. The health care industry has therefore been considering the feasibility of applying this methodology to its own teamwork-building and patient safety–promoting efforts.

Some organizations have been applying the CRM methodology in the operating room by describing the team performance inputs that are critical to essential team functions that, in turn, lead to desired outcomes (defined as patient well-being). Examples of inputs include individual aptitudes, physical environment, and culture (professional, organizational, and national). Performance functions consist of team formation and management, surgical procedures, communications, decision processes, and situational awareness.[5]

Another application of CRM to the health environment is the *MedTeams Behavior-Based Teamwork System,* developed by Dynamics Research Corporation, located in Andover, Massachusetts, and sponsored by the Army Research Laboratory. This system has been applied through courses and assessment tools and includes five team dimensions or goals: maintain team structure and climate, facilitate planning and problem solving, enhance communication among team members, facilitate workload management, and improve team-building skills. Each goal is tied to specific teamwork tasks. For example, tasks for the first goal (maintain team structure and climate) include "establish team leader," "form the team," "set team goals," and "assign roles and responsibilities." This approach is based on avoiding errors, trapping errors as they occur, and mitigating the consequences of errors. The following principles underlie the MedTeams approach:

- Team responsibility for patients

- A belief in clinician fallibility
- Peer monitoring
- Team member awareness of patient status, team member status, and institutional resources[6]

Some health care organizations are applying the CRM approach to their team-building efforts, with positive results to date. "We have been using CRM as our team-building strategy for some time now, and it has been showing some positive results as far as helping us define a specific team structure and allowing the whole team to fulfill their roles and bring up any real patient safety concerns," notes Lawrence Shuer, M.D., chief medical officer of Stanford Hospital and Clinics and Lucile Packard Children's Hospital, Stanford, CA. Shuer points to use of the methodology as one of the various ways by which organizations are ensuring and promoting patient safety and a culture of safety. "We have also devised our code of conduct and process to deal with disruptive behavior for the same reason: We have no tolerance in our institution for any process that could impair patient safety or negatively impact our work environment," he continues.

Communication

The Joint Commission has identified communication as the leading root cause of sentinel events in health care organizations. A breakdown in communication can lead to misunderstandings and mishaps, and this happens all too often in health care organizations. In order to get the message across to staff of the imperative for improved communication in the organization, a five-step process can be followed to help staff understand and embrace the new approach:

- *Step 1: Develop a clear and consistent organizationwide message regarding patient safety.* If everyone has a common understanding, and if the message is continually reinforced in all areas and levels of the organization, staff will begin to incorporate it into their daily activities. Communication about this issue should be constant, consistent, and delivered through diverse channels so that all staff can be reached.
- *Step 2: Link effective communication to patient safety.* If staff see concrete, justifiable reasons behind the drive to improve communication, and if those reasons can be expressed in terms that resonate with staff, they will be more supportive of the cultural change. If staff consider the harmful consequences of poor communication (even as it relates to disruptive behavior), the cultural shift will gain support.

- *Step 3: Make changing the culture a team effort.* Although leadership support is critical to culture change, everyone must be on board for such a program to be successful. Educating staff on the value of communication, as well as providing team training and other communication training programs, can help empower the staff to change. All members of the organization should be held accountable for communication improvement.
- *Step 4: Set the tone for an open and honest culture.* All the training in the world will not help change a culture if staff are blamed and punished for reporting errors and speaking up about safety concerns, including if they are penalized or retaliated against for filing a complaint about disruptive behavior. Conversations between leadership and staff should reinforce this concept. Also, leadership should lead by example: if leadership is using effective communication techniques, their example will resonate with staff.
- *Step 5: Communicate through multiple channels.* People communicate in a variety of ways, and different situations require different types of communication. For example, the way an organization communicates with staff about a new policy is different from the way a physician communicates with a nurse about a patient's care. Training can help educate staff on the different (and appropriate) ways to communicate.[7]

In his work training physicians on how to respond more appropriately to a staff member who is questioning an order without having an outburst or other disruptive reaction, Bill Swiggart, M.A., teaches a phrase that helps physicians be responsive and less disruptive "I teach them to say 'You might be right,'" he explains. It lets them acknowledge the concern expressed by the staff member while allowing them time to think about the question without having a negative reaction or being rude. Swiggart has observed that the physicians he has worked with have found this to be a particularly effective phrase.

In Sidebar 4-2 on pages 73–74, John-Henry Pfifferling, Ph.D., shares how the Center for Professional Well-Being mentors and trains staff through a process to establish professional behaviors. A big part of the center's process of helping deal with disruptive behavior is training physicians on how to communicate appropriately and more effectively with those around them. The principles in Sidebar 4-2 can be applied to other staff who may also need to learn some core principles related to effective communication.

Sidebar 4-2
Professional Behaviors

These are items Center for Professional Well-Being facilitators use in setting up criteria for professionalism (effective interprofessional communication to foster positive outcomes).

1. After a discussion or a presentation on the relationship between professionalism and the nobility of medicine, begin your homework as below.

2. **Rewrite** or use these behavioral descriptors to initiate a professionalism guide ("Professionalism Compact") for your practice/hospital or organization.

   The outcome can be a compact, with a signed pledge incorporated as a by-laws item, associated with **appropriate rewards (affirmations) and/or sanctions.**

   This guide is a covenant articulating professionalism criteria.

3. We propose that individuals assign some priorities to separate items and then meet in facilitated groups (within or across specialties) to craft a feasible **pilot** document.

4. After a "season" of experimentation with the pilot document (where we expect discussion of how the guide is shaping up), craft your refined list into a compact and consider **requiring a signature** from all credentialed professionals.

5. Incorporate the guide in your professional well-being program. Such a compact, when monitored, will prevent nearly all, but not all, conflict associated with allegations and management of disruptive behavior.

6. Incorporate other health professionals in the compact as the institution progresses in its professionalism program. Results can then become merged as a core component of culture-building in an institution.

Sanctions are a related and more complicated issue. Sanctions when someone violates compact principles need to be managed in focused and ongoing professional evaluations and performance review. Due process, due diligence, and fairness standards with an appeals process needs to be built into your system. Regular training and upgrading of content in conflict resolution and constructive feedback techniques are other essential components of a professionalism commitment.

The following are phrases and behaviors for your use:

- Clearly explain the basis for decisions.
- Use well-reasoned arguments to support proposals.
- Use well-reasoned arguments to support counter-proposals.
- Offer well-reasoned counter-arguments when you disagree.
- Openly provide information that others might not have.
- Admit your concerns for any "mistakes."
- Express your empathy for the consequences of "mistakes."
- Directly apologize when a "mistake" has occurred.
- Express plans to correct and/or prevent future "mistakes."
- Offer suggestions that get right to the point.
- Tell others clearly what you want.
- Offer suggestions that build on others' ideas.
- State your needs and expectations reasonably.
- Keep others' attention on issues you feel are important.
- Offer mutually beneficial exchanges and incentives.
- Express appreciation when someone does something well.
- Express your dissatisfaction when someone doesn't do something well.
- Tell others what you like about what they are doing.
- Tell others what you don't like about what they are doing.
- Gracefully accept feedback.
- Describe possibilities in ways that encourage others to share enthusiasm and commitment.
- Use images and vivid descriptions to heighten others' enthusiasm about possibilities.
- Stress the importance of pulling together to achieve a common vision/goals.
- Talk from the heart about values and ideals using "I" language.
- Encourage others to do more than they thought was possible.
- Give the time and attention others need to get their point across.
- Pay careful attention—without interrupting—when someone is trying to make a point.
- Focus carefully on concerns that someone else expresses.
- Back off if the timing is not right.
- Face up to important issues and help move them toward resolution.

(continued)

Sidebar 4-2
Professional Behaviors, *continued*

- Remain patient and receptive when someone disagrees with or challenges your point of view.
- Ask for the basis of the other's decisions: "Help me understand how you (believe that?)."
- Ask others for suggestions.
- Ask questions such as, "Could you give me a few examples to help me understand?"
- Ask questions like, "How can I help?" or "How can I support you?"
- Focus on "What can we learn from this 'mistake'" not on "Who is to blame?"
- Ask directly about the effects your behavior has on someone else.
- Communicate your understanding by paraphrasing what you have been told.
- Act as a sounding board to help clarify others' thinking.
- Summarize areas of agreement or mutual interest.
- Try to clarify and explore points on which you differ or disagree.
- Communicate understanding through the tone of the voice.
- Communicate your understanding of how a situation makes others feel.
- Show your genuine desire to find out how someone else feels.
- Give your support when someone else is facing difficult situations.
- Give others the courage to disclose how they feel about themselves.
- Empathize with others (for example, "Hearing you describe what you've been through, I feel [sad, mad, angry, scared, frustrated].").

Comparable criteria to develop a practice culture of professionalism (respectful communication):

- We accept the pressure toward perfectionism but simultaneously acknowledge the reality that progress, not perfection, will secure collegiality.
- We will deal with conflict consciously, with a willingness to deal with (not run away from) conflict.
- Sarcasm and cynicism are not welcome in our communications; our words will, to the best of our abilities, be used to support and nourish others.
- We will not hold each other to impossible standards.
- We will not condemn each when they appear to be wrong but will use the incident as a learning event.
- We will guard against an atmosphere of judging others.
- We will not ignore distress among members of the practice, nor do we have to solve each person's problems.
- Anger, impatience, and annoyance will be used as a symptom to understand and promote tolerance and calm.
- Order and efficiency will not control our group's life.
- Automatically focusing on what is wrong will also serve as a symptom that imbalance has gained power.

Sources

1. Rubin I., Campbell T.: *The ABCs of Effective Feedback.* San Francisco: Jossey-Bass, 1998
2. Riso, D.R.: *Enneagram Transformations.* Boston: Houghton-Mifflin, 1993.
3. Pfifferling, J.-H. Burnout: Effectively managing a grief syndrome. *Being Well* 4(1–2):1–18, 2002.

In establishing an effective and consistent process to deal with disruptive behavior, you may find that the issue and solution cross over many areas of responsibility and can involve many staff in helping plan a solution. This should be viewed in a positive light. The more that staff become aware of the zero-tolerance approach to disruptive behavior, the more likely they will be to use alternative means to communicate concerns and play their part to ensure that the organization nurtures a respectful, encouraging, and open environment where disruptive behavior has no place.

Don't forget to celebrate the accomplishments and the transformation you will observe as these qualities and principles become firmly ingrained in the culture of the organization, a culture that is safety focused.

 ## For Your Consideration

1. This chapter delineates the steps that can be taken to establish a process to deal with disruptive behavior. What steps has your organization taken and what steps does it still need to take? What has proven particularly effective? What has been particularly ineffective?

2. What training and education processes do you have in place related to improving communication and teamwork? What methodologies do you use? What do you think will be most effective in helping develop these skills among your organization's staff?

In addition to ensuring that there is a code of conduct that delineates disruptive and acceptable behavior and developing and implementing a process to deal with disruptive behavior effectively, organizations should plan to train and empower staff to respond and work to resolve any disruptive events as they take place. Chapter 5 offers suggestions on and strategies for using conflict resolution and other approaches to deal with disruptive behavior.

References

1. Lin D.: Why every hospital should have a code of conduct. *Focus on Patient Safety* 7(2):4–5, 2004.

2. Porto G., Lauve R.: Disruptive clinician behavior: A persistent threat to patient safety. *Patient Saf Qual Healthc* 3(4):16–24, 2006.

3. Temple University Hospital: *Physicians' Health Committee.* http://www.temple.edu/tuhphc/QandA.htm (accessed Apr. 14, 2007).

4. Pizzi L., Goldfarb N., Nash D.: *Crew Resource Management and Its Applications in Medicine.* http://www.ahrq.gov/clinic/ptsafety/pdf/chap44.pdf (accessed Apr. 14, 2007).

5. Helmreich R.L., Schaefer H.G.: Team performance in the operating room. In Bogner M.S. (ed.): *Human Error in Medicine.* Hillside, NJ: Lawrence Erlbaum, 1998.

6. Risser D.T., et al.: The potential for improved teamwork to reduce medical errors in the emergency department. The MedTeams Research Consortium. *Ann Emerg Med* 34:373–383, 1999.

7. Joint Commission Resources: *The Joint Commission Guide to Improving Staff Communication.* Oakbrook Terrace, IL: The Joint Commission, 2005.

Chapter 5

Toward a Culture of Safety:
Conflict Resolution and Other Approaches to Preventing Disruptive Behavior

> **In this chapter:** This chapter provides tools and tips organizations can use to empower employees to defuse conflict and regain a healthy working relationship. This chapter also provides helpful resources and information on a number of national health care initiatives that promote healthy work environments, excellence, and a culture of safety. In addition, this chapter provides a number of scenarios, as well as strategies and tips on how to approach each of those scenarios based on the topics and material covered throughout this publication.

Building a culture of safety is a necessity in health care organizations. An important building block in the process of establishing a culture of safety is ensuring that negative behaviors and activities, such as disruptive behavior, are eliminated from the status quo of the organization. In addition to drafting and implementing a code of conduct and a process to deal with disruptive behavior, an organization can integrate certain techniques and processes into its structure to help establish that culture. Staff can be educated on and trained to use conflict reduction or resolution techniques to help them on a day-to-day basis. Conflict resolution is an effective way to deal with disruptive behavior, among other things. This chapter looks at conflict resolution and other techniques that can be used to help staff deal with disruptive behavior.

Conflict Resolution

Conflict resolution builds stronger, more cohesive organizations and more rewarding relationships. Resolving a conflict and moving on to a successful working relationship is both difficult and necessary.

Conflict resolution refers to a wide range of processes that encourage nonviolent dispute resolution outside the traditional court system. The field of conflict resolution also includes efforts in schools and communities to reduce violence and bullying and aid in the development of communication and problem-solving skills. The following are some common forms of conflict resolution:

- **Negotiation:** A discussion among two or more people, with the goal of reaching an agreement.
- **Mediation:** A voluntary and confidential process in which a neutral third-party facilitator helps people discuss difficult issues and negotiate an agreement. Basic steps in the process include gathering information, framing the issues, developing options, negotiating, and formalizing agreements. Parties in mediation create their own solutions, and the mediator does not have any decision-making power over the outcome.
- **Arbitration:** A process in which a neutral third party, after reviewing evidence and listening to arguments from both sides, issues a decision to settle the case. Arbitration is often used in commercial and labor/management disputes.
- **Mediation–arbitration:** A hybrid that combines mediation and arbitration. Before the session, the disputing parties agree to try mediation first but give the neutral third party the authority to make a decision if mediation is not successful.
- **Early neutral evaluation:** A process that involves using a court-appointed attorney to review a case before it goes to trial. The attorney reviews the merits of the case and encourages the parties to attempt resolution. If there is no resolution, the attorney informs the disputants about how to proceed with litigation and gives an opinion on the likely outcome if the case goes to trial.
- **Community conferencing:** A structured conversation involving all members of a community (offenders, victims, family, friends, and so on) who have been affected by a dispute or a crime. Using a script, the facilitator invites people to express how they were affected and how they wish to address and repair the harm that resulted.
- **Collaborative law:** A process for solving disputes in which attorneys commit to reaching a settlement without using litigation.

- **Negotiated rule making:** A collaborative process in which government agencies seek input from a variety of stakeholders before issuing a new rule.
- **Peer mediation:** A process in which people act as mediators to help resolve disputes among their peers.[1]

What Types of Disputes Can Be Addressed Through Conflict Resolution?

Conflict resolution can be used to help resolve almost any type of dispute within and outside the work environment. In the work environment, however, the types of conflicts that can be resolved in this manner include workplace disputes, policy issues, and health care disputes, among others.

Use of Conflict Resolution in Health Care

For a heath care organization that provides care, treatment, and services to those who can have multiple and complex needs, input from a number of health care disciplines and staff is often needed, and, effective teamwork is therefore essential. It has been noted, however, that the majority of those working in health care begin their professions with little or no formal teamwork training, including conflict resolution, in their discipline-specific education program. Teamwork training seems to occur through on-the-job experience.[2]

The response to conflict can occur in different ways. With a positive response, individuals take the time and effort to resolve conflict or preempt situations that may result in conflict; in a manipulative response, individuals maneuver situations in order to have an advantage when decisions are made; and in a negative response, a conflict is addressed by outright rejection of an opinion.

The Institute for Safe Medication Practices (ISMP) suggests the implementation of a conflict resolution process for staff involved in a conflict to "communicate effectively and protect patients, not to punish, embarrassed involved staff." It goes on to stress the need to ensure that the process "provides an avenue for resolution outside the typical chain of command if the conflict involves a subordinate and his supervisor. Following a 'two challenge rule' is one option. Used in highly reliable industries with excellent safety records, the rule requires communication of critical information twice to the same person. If there's no resolution, the matter is automatically referred to at least one other person before a final decision is made."[3] In the case of health care organizations, conflict resolution can be a helpful technique to address issues such as staff tension, disruptive behavior, organization structure, change management, and staffing changes. See the "For Your Consideration" box on pages 79–80 for an example of a scenario in which conflict resolution became an essential step in resolving tension in a medical clinic.

Applying and Learning Conflict Resolution

One way to train staff on using conflict resolution is to use a fun and unusual approach. Sometimes a fun activity can be an effective means to get a message across and also help the staff involved to form better connections with each other as they develop team-building skills. The following example provides one kind of conflict resolving game that can be played among staff. It may be a good idea to choose a non-health care–related topic (something amusing like "chocolate is good for you") initially to break the ice and get participants used to the idea of playing a game to learn conflict resolution skills. Once staff feel more comfortable with the methodology and approach, it is then a good idea to choose a topic that is closer to the workplace, such as collaboration on the health care team.

The Conflict Resolution Network

The Conflict Resolution Network (CRN) was founded in 1973 (then as a Peace Program of the United Nations Association of Australia). Its purpose is to research, develop, teach, and implement the theory and practice of conflict resolution at the national and international levels. Believing skills and structures for conflict resolution are transferable, CRN works with conflict whose nature is personal, community, workplace, or global. More information, including additional free conflict resolution–related resources, is available at http://www.crnhq.org.

Conflict resolution can be an effective way to defuse disruptive behavior or to teach staff ways to deal with such behavior as it happens. If there are no staff in the organization who can help facilitate training on conflict resolution, then it may be worthwhile to bring in external experts to walk staff through some conflict resolution techniques. This can go a long way toward helping to empower staff to deal directly and immediately with any disruptive situations.

For Your Consideration

Consider the following example:
The physician members of a gastroenterology clinic were struggling with how they wanted to approach call on the weekends. While all the members agreed that call should be rotated, some of the members felt that the rotation was not always fair because three of the physicians would find themselves occasionally called in on additional weekends because they could perform an additional procedure that the others could not.

After repeated group meetings to try to resolve the issue, the physicians were still not able to come to an agreement. Some physicians felt that the times that the physicians with the additional proficiency were called in were infrequent enough that it did not warrant a special accommodation and others felt that those who were called in should be compensated in some way, be it with additional time off during their own call weekend or some other arrangement. Other physicians felt concerned that that kind of arrangement would be too complicated and resource intensive to keep track of.

All the while, the physicians were growing ever more frustrated with the lack of resolution, and this tension was beginning to affect the work environment. On a Monday morning after a call weekend when one of the physicians who was not on call had been called in to handle the additional procedure that the physician on call could not handle, the physician who had been called in was exhibiting annoyance, frustration, and impatience, and staff were taking pains to have as little interaction with him as possible. Two nurses had already been on the receiving end of impatient outbursts and rude comments. When the physician saw another physician who had been very vocal at the practice meetings in saying that there was no real need to compensate the physicians who put in extra time, he erupted vocally at him, expressing his anger at "how absurd and unfair" the call rotation was and how he had missed his daughter's soccer game.

"I'm sick and tired of being treated like my time means less than anyone else's," he snapped at the physician before throwing down the chart he was holding and storming off. Because of the noise and publicity of the outburst, all of the clinic staff knew what had happened, including the clinic's manager. As a result, she approached clinic leadership to explain the situation and shared the troubles that the group was having coming to consensus about how to handle call fairly and in a way that would meet the needs of the whole group.

The clinic's leadership met with the physicians involved, and in turn met with the rest of the physicians in the clinic. It was clear that there was an inability for the group to come to a consensus without help. Leadership brought in conflict resolution specialists to hold a series of meetings with the physicians to help them resolve the issue in a fair manner and to prevent the possibility of the work environment growing dysfunctional or unhealthy for all of the staff.

When the mediation specialists came to the clinic, they worked in advance with the clinic manager to set up an agenda for the meeting. In the meeting, they took the following steps:
- The mediators asked each physician, "What do you think the problem is?" A mediator took notes to recap the answers.
- They asked each individual to share his or her point of view on call and what he or she thought the process should be. They asked everyone to "shoot for the moon" at first, and the others at the table were not to comment or react to what was being shared. One of the mediators took notes.
- When the requests were on the table, the mediators asked the participants to share what they felt was reasonable in the requests and what seemed unfair. This was also documented.
- Finally, the mediators asked the physicians to share any times that they felt personally affected (positively and negatively) by the call schedule.

The sharing process opened up a lot of eyes. It was not that these thoughts had not been shared before, but it was more that they were being shared in a way that required everyone to listen and learn. In addition, the physicians began to
(continued)

For Your Consideration, *continued*

understand why changes in call had been difficult for everyone. Those who lacked the training felt badly about having to call in other physicians, and those who had to come in felt their time was not as valued. And those who had come in for extra duties had been feeling the pressure at home as well. "My daughter was devastated when I missed the soccer game," the physician who had had the inappropriate outburst explained.

After more discussion, it was learned that the physicians who were called in more frequently to cover the extra procedure put in coverage on approximately one month extra per year. The physician who had called in that physician made a suggestion that he would be willing to cover call on one extra weekend a year for one of the physicians who would find himself called in more frequently as long as he would be available as a backup call physician on one of his call weekends. After the rest of the physician group agreed to this, they took time to map out the schedule for the rest of the year. What this meant was that the physicians who were not trained in

the additional procedure took on one more call weekend each year than the physicians who were trained, and those physicians who were trained divvied up the call weekend on which they could be called in by the non-trained physicians.

The physicians agreed to this approach, with the stipulation that they meet again in six months to reassess whether the new schedule was working.

1. Review this scenario and list the limiting factors that were making it impossible for the physician group to work through the issue effectively. Would you have done anything differently?
2. In this scenario, one of the issues appeared to be a lack of empathy to how the process was affecting each member of the group. Strategize ways to develop a firmer sense of empathy and respect for fellow staff in the work environment.

Lessons Learned: Tips and Strategies for Dealing with Disruptive Staff Members and Work Environments

Earlier in this chapter and in the preceding chapters, a number of real-life and reality-based scenarios have been presented for consideration to illustrate certain components of disruptive behavior. Paired with many of them are the varied approaches and strategies to deal with the kind of behavior taking place. The following is an additional scenario paired with suggested strategies for how to approach it. In addition, worksheet space is provided in Table 5-1 for you to map out scenarios from your own organization's experience and unique challenges.

Scenario 1

Providing excellent care was of paramount importance to Dr. Julie Smith. Her perception of life was that her work came first, and all else came after. Her focus was

so specific that it was often hard for her to understand why others may not have the same point of view. She was a perfectionist as well and was often anxious (although she held this inwardly) about making a mistake. Because she could not guarantee that those who worked around her were as committed or "perfect" as she was, she was often anxious about errors. Dr Smith's heavy focus on work and perfection often led her to bring issues to the attention of nursing leadership. She was often critical—though not rude—about what she felt were mistakes or problems among the nursing staff. And to her, all these issues were significant, though to the weary staff, it just felt like minutia. She was often a dreaded physician for new nurses to work with. As a result, staff were uncomfortable and intimidated around the doctor, and after a series of new nurses refused to work with her again, the nurse manager brought her concerns to leadership.

Issues

The physician's need for perfection and her own fear of failing has led her to become hypercritical of those around her, which has led staff to dread interactions with her. While her actions are not overly disruptive (no egregious abuse or harassment), they are disruptive enough that staff have begun reporting feeling worried that they will make mistakes due to feeling anxious while working with her.

Strategies for a Solution

Consider the following steps in planning a solution:

- In a situation such as this, an important element to keep in mind is that some work styles can be disruptive to other staff, but this does not mean that different work styles can't work effectively together.
- Leadership should investigate the issue closely and quickly to determine the root of the problem and what, if any, resources should be employed to help diffuse the situation.
- At this point, it is also important to collect any data or documentation on specific events that have taken place. It is more likely that having specific and documented material will resonate more effectively with those involved.
- Based on what is learned, a response should be put in place quickly. This should be in the form of a plan, and all affected parties should be involved.
- The use of specific staff resources for mediation, additional training, or teamwork building may be warranted. It may also be helpful to require that the physician undergo some one-on-one mentoring with an organization leader or an effective communications consultant to help her learn how to relay legitimate valid concerns (not minutia) and also how to prioritize the essential patient safety–related concerns versus minutia. What should be stressed is the fact that while the feedback on concerns is always welcome to staff, the crucial element that may need to be worked on is how that feedback is communicated. If these measures are ineffective, the plan in place should note escalation measures—such as mandatory anger management sessions or additional training on interpersonal skills.
- Staff should be offered training in effective communication techniques and mentored in conflict resolution so they can address concerns as they emerge.

For Your Consideration

1. Have you used methodologies such as conflict resolution in your organization before? What happened? How effective was it?
2. Does anyone in your organization possess conflict management or resolution skills? If not, what steps can you take to send a staff member for training or to bring in an outside expert to train staff?

Use Table 5-1 on page 84 to map out the types of situations that have taken palce or are taking place in your organization, highlight the issues or problems that are inherent in the situation, and brainstorm some strategies for how to resolve the situation.

In any given situation, a number of strategies may exist, and a variety of options may present themselves. Most important of all is ensuring that whatever strategy is employed should be clearly documented, faithfully and consistently followed through, and involve all the necessary staff members. The strategy should also be focused on successfully assisting all staff involved in finding a way to work together effectively and in a nondisruptive manner. There are, of course, instances in which a staff member's behavior is so egregious or detrimental that the only effective strategy is to terminate his or her interaction with the organization.

National Initiatives to Help Improve Work Environments and Team Skills

Throughout the health care field, there are new methodologies and initiatives in place to promote healthy work environments, improved staffing conditions, and a culture of safety mind-set. Some of these have been explored in previous chapters, but in the following two examples, we see how two national nursing associations are attempting to address the issue of moving toward a culture of safety in different ways. In the case of the "Magnet hospital" approach, by rewarding hospitals with this designation for improving collaboration and communication among staff, these hospitals are actually seeing an improvement in the quality and safety of care, treatment, and services being delivered.

Sidebar 5-1
An Expert Perspective: Using Conflict Resolution in Health Care

Note: A number of years ago, Leonard Marcus, Ph.D., director of the program for health care negotiation and conflict resolution at the Harvard School of Public Health, was interviewed in *Physician Executive* magazine about his thoughts on the need for and the use of conflict resolution in health care. The following are some excerpts from that article to provide some perspective on how conflict resolution can function in health care.

While conflict can be destructive, it also can provide opportunities for people to look at where there are problems, to identify and correct those problems, and end up on the other side with something even better than what they began with. We are hoping that people will recognize the opportunity to turn problems into solutions and that the book provides guidance in that effort.

I think the greatest benefit to finding methods for collaboration would be in better accomplishing what we are all committed to in the health care system. That is not to say that there won't be conflicts and differences of opinion, but that those conflicts will focus our attention on how to build improvements. The intent is not to say that we will always agree on everything, but rather that when a conflict or difference of opinion does occur, it not be the cause for war or the escalation of our disputes. It is really a matter of saying let's sit down, have a way of constructively discussing these issues and differences, and figure out how we can move forward.

We always say that the product of negotiation can be only as good as the process used to come up with its result. . . . People can get so caught up in the conflict that they can't even see the costs of escalation and the potential benefits of resolution.

[I stress] the importance of looking at a problem from different perspectives. Many times, when we're mediating a dispute, if we ask one person about the problem, they give us one definition. We turn to the other person and hear a completely different definition. And we say, no wonder you can't solve "the problem," you are both bringing different problems to the table.

We teach people the methods of negotiation and conflict resolution, multidimensional problem-solving, and the process that we have developed called the "Walk in the Woods." It is not only a matter of hearing lectures and learning in a didactic way. In fact, most of the week-long course is focused on interactive negotiation exercises and simulations. People conduct simulated mediations in front of a video camera and are critiqued. It is very much hands-on.

. . . one of the things that we say is as a negotiator or as a mediator, what you do, what you say, how you are perceived is part of the tool of your negotiation. As a negotiator or a mediator you are constantly being observed and assessed and we give people an understanding of what others are seeing, what messages they are sending, and what they themselves need to perceive and understand.

If you are about to drive your family over a bridge, you would like to think that the people who poured the concrete, laid the steel beams, and constructed the road that led up to it were working together in harmony, so that the bridge does what it was intended to do. Similarly, in the health care system, if someone comes to us for care, they have the expectation that we have the same level of coordination, cooperation, and collaboration in our work. And even though there are many difficult issues that are facing us—financial, professional, and organizational—we still must maintain that commitment to work together.

Source: Based on Reece R.L.: *Renegotiating health care: an interview with Leonard Marcus, Ph.D.—Conflict Management—Interview. Physician Exec* 25(4), 1999. Reprinted with permission.

Marcus's Approach to Conflict Resolution in Health Care

The Health Care Negotiation and Conflict Resolution program at the Harvard School of Public Health, led by Leonard Marcus, teaches a four-step process for conflict resolution:

Step 1: Self-Interests

Each participant articulates his or her view of key problems, issues, and options. All participants are encouraged to actively listen, question, and interact with one another.

Step 2: Enlarged Interests

The participants reframe their understanding of current problems and possible options with a wider perspective, based on the integrative listening and confidence-building that occurred in step 1.

Step 3: Enlightened Interests

The group is ready to engage in innovative thinking and problem solving, generating ideas and perspectives that had not previously been considered.

Step 4: Aligned Interests

Participants build common-ground perspectives, priorities, action items, agreement, or plans for moving forward. Depending on the scope of the intended objectives, at this point, they recognize the tangible contributions and opportunities accomplished through the meeting.

The Magnet Hospital Approach:

Improved Communication and Collaboration Among Staff

The Magnet hospital approach is gaining wide acclaim and attention as an effective program initiated by the American Nurses Credentialing Center (ANCC) to recognize health care organizations that provide nursing excellence. The program also provides a vehicle for disseminating successful nursing practices and strategies. In the words of the ANCC:

> Recognizing quality patient care, nursing excellence, and innovations in professional nursing practice, the Magnet Recognition Program provides consumers with the ultimate benchmark to measure the quality of care that they can expect to receive. When *U.S. News & World Report* publishes its annual showcase of "America's Best Hospitals," being a Nurse Magnet™ facility contributes to the total score for quality of inpatient care. Of the 14 medical centers listed on the exclusive Honor Roll with the 2006 rankings (as of July 17, 2006), 7 of the top 10 were Magnet hospitals.

The Magnet Recognition Program is based on quality indicators and standards of nursing practice as defined in the American Nurses Association's Scope and Standards for Nurse Administrators (2004). The Scope and Standards for Nurse Administrators and other "foundational documents" form the base upon which the Magnet environment is built. The Magnet designation process includes the appraisal of qualitative factors in nursing. These factors, referred to as "Forces of Magnetism" were first identified through research done in 1983.

The full expression of the forces embodies a professional environment guided by a strong visionary nursing leader who advocates and supports development and excellence in nursing practice. As a natural outcome of this, the program elevates the reputation and standards of the nursing profession.[5]

Table 5-1. Disruptive Behavior Situations with Issues and Strategy Planning

Scenario/Situation	Issues	Strategies

For Your Consideration

1. Try out the Conflict Resolving Game, pages 86–88, with five other colleagues or members of the leadership team. What were your observations and what did you learn about your own conflict resolution skills? How can you incorporate conflict resolution into your organization?

American Association for Critical Care Nurses' Healthy Work Environment Initiative: Its Vision for the Future

In 2005, the American Association of Critical-Care Nurses (AACN) released a set of six standards that it believes must be met in order for a work environment to be "healthy." These standards outline crucial staffing and cultural elements that resonate with the kind of work environment needed to defuse disruptive behavior. They speak to skilled communication, collaboration, authentic leadership, appropriate staffing, meaningful recognition, and effective decision making. Excerpts from the AACN's 2005 publication, *AACN Standards for Establishing and Sustaining Healthy Work Environments: A Journey to Excellence* have been reprinted in the Appendix with permission.

This document provides a blueprint of sorts that should be taken into consideration when establishing and developing a healthy work environment. The qualities stressed in the document should be at the forefront of the organization's mind when it plans and improves its own work environment, particularly when it works to heal the damage in a toxic work environment caused by disruptive behavior. Reviewing this publication can provide some helpful examples of how staff should interact with each other.

Conclusion

Much of this publication has been about negative behavior that has poisoned the well-being and safety of health care organizations for years and how it has affected organizations and their staff in countless ways. The publication has also offered strategies and tips on ways to cope with that unacceptable behavior. The examples provided in this chapter point to where organizations now need to go: to a patient-safe environment, to a culture of safety, and to truly establishing a civil work atmosphere that has no room for disruptive behavior. In order to really make the

vision of a culture of safety come to life in an organization, disruptive behavior and its detrimental, divisive, and demoralizing effects must cease to exist.

Perhaps the most poignant reminder of the need and imperative to remove an antithesis to a culture of safety such as disruptive behavior from the workplace are the words of Charles Schwab:

I have yet to find the man, however exalted his station, who did not do better work and put forth greater effort under a spirit of approval than under a spirit of criticism.

While Schwab may not have been speaking specifically about health care, his words resonate as a reminder that demonstrating qualities such as civility, kindness, encouragement, dignity, and respect in the workplace can truly inspire staff toward greatness.

The delivery of safe, high-quality care does not happen in a vacuum. It happens in the midst of a busy health care environment that is rich with complexity, varied cultures, different work styles, and differerent personalities and skills. The ideal of achieving a safe, high-quality, civil work environment where people feel respected, appreciated, heard, and valued is not out of reach. With systematic, consistent efforts to put in place policies, procedures, and processes that clearly map out a code of conduct and list of expectations for all staff, eventually the mindset will shift, and a culture of safety will come to life for the benefit of staff, patients, and the community at large.

References

1. Association for Conflict Resolution: *Frequently Asked Questions About Conflict Resolution.* http://www.acrnet.org/about/CR-FAQ.htm (accessed Jun. 6, 2007).
2. Curtin-Telegdi N.: *Conflict Resolution: The Good, the Bad, and the Ugly: Experiences of Chronic Care Hospital Team Members.* http://www.ahs.uwaterloo.ca/~cahr/news/vol18/conflict.html (accessed Jun. 6, 2007).
3. Institute for Safe Medication Practices: Intimidation: Practitioners speak up about this unresolved problem (Part I). *ISMP Medication Safety Alert* Mar. 11, 2004.
4. Reece, R.L.: Renegotiating health care: An interview with Leonard Marcus, Ph.D.—Conflict Management—Interview. *Physician Exec.* 25(4) , 1999.
5. American Nurses Credentialing Center: *What Is the Magnet Recognition Program?* http://nursecredentialing.org/magnet/ (accessed Jun. 7, 2007).

Guidelines for Playing the Conflict Resolving Game

Purpose

In the Conflict Resolving Game, participants address an issue with the purpose of resolving some of the conflicts within it.

An additional purpose is to learn and practice the skills of conflict resolution in order to use these skills in real-life situations.

Choosing the Issue

Choose an issue and word it in a neutral way. Instead of "Is the government adequately addressing the problems of unemployed youth?" (which calls for a "yes" or "no" answer), use unbiased language like: "What can be done to ease the problem of youth unemployment?" (which leaves it open-ended). Once the issue is well worded, look for the specific conflict areas that can be raised under it (for example, staff retention, competency, and patient safety).

Some Suggested Issues for Focus

In your choice of topic, undoubtedly you will be influenced by interest and information availability. Try to choose topics in which you know there is conflict. Here are some current issues to consider:

- **Personal experience:** Job training, staff safety, health care worker safety
- **Community concern:** Emergency management, infection control issues/epidemics, staff retention and/or training
- **Global significance:** Patient safety, medication management.

The Facilitator

The facilitator needs to read this document to be familiar with the guidelines and tools of the Conflict Resolving Game. (In a classroom situation, the teacher may play the role of facilitator.)

The facilitator's role could include coaching, assessing, inviting audience participation, suggesting topics, and referring to relevant conflict resolution resources. The facilitator need not perform all these roles but may choose to adopt one or more.

A facilitator might also assist team preparation and audience involvement by handing out, ahead of time, a list of some specific conflicts within the chosen issue. The facilitator may involve the audience in discussion and question time, between speakers, at the end, or both. The facilitator could follow the evolving problem-solving closely, summarizing and seeking clarification of each speaker's key points.

Format

By prior agreement, each player can speak independently or belong to a team.

There are many ways to play the Conflict Resolving Game. You might try two teams with three players each.

The facilitator could select speakers for each team or some speakers may be able to elect themselves to the team of their choice. The facilitator usually decides which team begins. Then speakers alternate, one from each team. A good guideline is no interruptions, one person speaking at a time.

Each team represents the perspective of one party involved. For instance, in the issue "what can be done to ease the problem of youth unemployment?" one team could represent unemployed youth, and the other could represent government.

Participants Are Conflict Resolvers

Each speaker is called a conflict resolver and is addressed by that title throughout the game (for example, "The second conflict resolver to speak will be . . ."; "Analysis of the issue will be done by the first conflict resolver, . . .", "Would all conflict resolvers join their own team for five minutes' strategy conference?") Conflict resolvers may speak with or without notes; spontaneity and preparation are equally valued.

Assessment

The Conflict Resolving Game is a new concept of winning. Success is everyone gaining something from the proposed solution(s). Therefore, the game may be played with or

(continued)

Guidelines for Playing the Conflict Resolving Game, *continued*

without point scoring. Individual or team scores may be announced.

Speakers may be assessed or scored on:
I. **Role tasks**—how well they perform their role (*see* "Role tasks")
II. **Competency-Based Assessment Criteria**—Judged by their ability to use appropriate conflict resolution skills (*see* "Competency-Based Assessment Criteria")

The facilitator only may score, or all listeners could have checklists to assess each speaker. The first time a group plays the game in teams, role tasks only might be issued for scoring.

A well-played conflict resolving game will perform three role tasks analyses, present options, and offer solutions.

I. Role Tasks
Use the following for a "two teams, each with three speakers" variation. If scoring, the facilitator may tick boxes or use a 1–5 grading, scoring the speaker only for the role he or she should be taking. Note: The parallels with first, second, and third speakers in traditional debates.

Conflict Resolver 1: Analysis
❐ Clearly state the conflicts seen from your team's point of view.
❐ Clearly state your team's needs and concerns regarding these conflicts.
❐ Do not offer solutions at this stage.

Conflict Resolver 2: Options
❐ Present the options and describe how they meet your team's needs and concerns.
❐ Be objective; don't be for or against any one option.
❐ Respond as a conflict resolver to the points made by earlier speakers.

Conflict Resolver 3: Solutions
❐ Put forward your team's solutions or action plan.

❐ Say why your suggestions work best for everyone and deal with any problems.
❐ Respond to earlier speakers on both teams.

Fouls
Players may lose points by:
Name-calling ❐
Stereotyping or making racist, agist, or sexist remarks ❐
Put-downs ❐
Blaming ❐
No acknowledgement of previous speaker's key point ❐
Threatening verbal or body language ❐
Interrupting ❐
Introducing irrelevancies ❐

I. Competency-Based Assessment Criteria
If scoring, tick boxes or use 1–5 grading. No speaker needs to demonstrate all 12 of the skills. Assess their ability to apply the relevant skills to appropriate contexts:

1. **Win—Win**
   ❐ Potential opponents are treated as problem-solving partners.
2. **Creative Response**
   ❐ Positive attitudes to addressing conflicts are displayed.
3. **Empathy**
   ❐ Speakers acknowledge the other team's point of view and add value to it.
4. **Appropriate Assertiveness**
   ❐ Without blaming or attacking, the team's own needs are clearly stated.
5. **Cooperative Power**
   ❐ Where power imbalance affects decision making, appropriate responses to the inequalities are defined.
6. **Managing Emotions**
   ❐ The speaker's emotions are expressed, and the other team's emotions are acknowledged.
7. **Willingness to Resolve**
   ❐ Benefits of resolving—for all parties—are developed.
8. **Mapping the Conflict**
   ❐ All key parties are identified, and their needs and concerns are outlined.

(continued)

Guidelines for Playing the Conflict Resolving Game, *continued*

9. Designing Options

❏ A wide range of options are considered, without debating or justifying at this stage.

10. Negotiation

❏ Fair, just, and commonsense offers are made.

11. Mediation

❏ The option of an impartial and objective third-party mediator is presented.

12. Broadening Perspectives

❏ Suggested solutions are presented in terms of how they affect the broader context beyond the issue itself.

Preparation

• Read this document and discuss it.

• Choose the issue, define the specific conflicts involved, and gather background information.

If playing with a team:

• Meet with your own team members to jointly prepare and agree on each speaker's key points.

• If time allows, rehearse together.

Preparation may be as little as 15 minutes (particularly for experienced players) or several weeks. Experiment and note the difference.

Source: http://www.crnhq.org/crgame.html. The Conflict Resolution Network © 2007. Used with permission.

American Association for Critical Care Nurses' Healthy Work Environment Initiative

Excerpt from *AACN Standards for Establishing and Sustaining Healthy Work Environments: A Journey to Excellence*

Each day, thousands of medical errors harm the patients and families served by the American health care system. Work environments that tolerate ineffective interpersonal relationships and do not support education to acquire necessary skills perpetuate unacceptable conditions. So do health professionals who experience moral distress over this state of affairs, yet remain silent and overwhelmed with resignation. Consider again these all-too-familiar situations:

- A nurse chooses not to call a physician known to be verbally abusive. The nurse uses her judgment to clarify a prescribed medication and administers a fatal dose of the wrong drug.
- Additional patients added to a nurse's assignment during a busy weekend because on-call staff is not available and back up plans do not exist to cover variations in patient census. Patients are placed at risk for errors and injury and nurses are frustrated and angry.
- Isolated decision-making in one department leads to tension, frustration and a higher risk of errors by all involved. Whether affecting patient care or unit operations, decisions made without including all parties places everyone involved at risk.
- Nurses placed in leadership positions without adequate preparation and support for their role. The resulting environment creates dissatisfaction and high turnover for nurse leaders and staff as well.
- Contentious relationships between nurses and administrators heightened when managers are required to stretch their responsibilities without adequate preparation and coaching for success. Only 65% of hospital managers are held accountable for employee satisfaction.

Each situation characterizes poor and ineffective relationships. Attention to work relationships is often dismissed as unworthy of resource allocation in health care today, especially when those resources are aimed at supporting education and development of essential skills. This is because of the mistaken perception that effective relationships do not affect an organization's financial health. Nothing could be further from the truth. Relationship issues are real obstacles to the development of work environments where patients and their families can receive safe, even excellent, care. Inattention to work relationships creates obstacles that may become the root cause of medical errors, hospital-acquired infections and other complications, patient readmission and nurse turnover.

Adequately addressing the reputedly "soft" issues that involve relationships is the key to halting the epidemic of treatment-related harm to patients and the continued erosion of the bottom line in health care organizations. Indeed, the Institute of Medicine has reported that safety and quality problems exist in large part because dedicated health professionals work within systems that neither prepare nor support them to achieve optimal patient care outcomes.

Addressing these issues aligns with nurses' ethical obligations. Specifically, the obligations to establish, maintain and improve health care environments and employment conditions conducive to providing quality care consistent with the values of the profession, and to maintain compassionate and caring relationships with "a commitment to fair treatment of individuals and integrity-preserving compromise."

Six Essential Standards

The American Association of Critical-Care Nurses (AACN) recognizes the inextricable links among quality of the work environment, excellent nursing practice and patient care outcomes. The AACN Synergy Model for Patient Care further affirms how excellent nursing practice is that which meets the needs of patients and their families.

AACN is strategically committed to bringing its influence and resources to bear on creating work and care environments that are safe, healing, humane and respectful of the rights, responsibilities, needs and contributions of all people—including patients, their families and nurses.

Six standards for establishing and sustaining healthy work environments have been identified. The standards represent evidence-based and relationship-centered principles of professional performance. Each standard is considered essential since studies show that effective and sustainable outcomes do not emerge when any standard is considered optional.

The standards align directly with the core competencies for health professionals recommended by the Institute of Medicine. They support the education of all health professionals "to deliver patient-centered care as members of an interdisciplinary team, emphasizing evidence-based practice, quality improvement approaches, and informatics." With these standards, AACN contributes to the implementation of elements in a healthy work environment articulated in 2004 by the 70-member Nursing Organizations Alliance.

The standards further support the education of nurse leaders to acquire the core competencies of self-knowledge, strategic vision, risk-taking and creativity, interpersonal and communication effectiveness, and inspiration identified by the Robert Wood Johnson Executive Nurse Fellows Program.

The standards are neither detailed nor exhaustive. They do not address dimensions such as physical safety, clinical practice, clinical and academic education and credentialing, all of which are amply addressed by a multitude of statutory, regulatory and professional agencies and organizations.

The standards are designed to be used as a foundation for thoughtful reflection and engaged dialogue about the current realities of each work environment. Critical elements required for successful implementation accompany each standard. Working collaboratively, individuals and groups within an organization should determine the priority and depth of application required to implement each standard.

The standards for establishing and sustaining healthy work environments are:

Skilled Communication
Nurses must be as proficient in communication skills as they are in clinical skills.

True Collaboration
Nurses must be relentless in pursuing and fostering true collaboration.

Effective Decision Making
Nurses must be valued and committed partners in making policy, directing and evaluating clinical care and leading organizational operations.

Appropriate Staffing
Staffing must ensure the effective match between patient needs and nurse competencies.

Meaningful Recognition
Nurses must be recognized and must recognize others for the value each brings to the work of the organization.

Authentic Leadership
Nurse leaders must fully embrace the imperative of a healthy work environment, authentically live it and engage others in its achievement.

Standard 1: Skilled Communication
Nurses must be as proficient in communication skills as they are in clinical skills.

Optimal care of patients mandates that the specialized knowledge and skills of nurses, physicians, administrators and multiple other professionals be integrated. This integration will be accomplished only through frequent, respectful interaction and skilled communication. Skilled communication is more than the one-way delivery of information; it is a two-way dialogue in which people think and decide together.

A culture of safety and excellence requires that individual nurses and health care organizations make it a priority to develop among professionals communication skills—including written, spoken and non-verbal—that are on a par with expert clinical skills. This culture expects civility and respects nurses who speak from their knowledge and authority.

Patients in the care of clinically expert professionals suffer medical errors with alarming frequency. Nearly 3 in 4 errors are caused by human factors associated with interpersonal interactions. In addition, according to data from The Joint Commission, breakdown in team communication is a top contributor to sentinel events.

Intimidating behavior and deficient interpersonal relationships lead to mistrust, chronic stress and dissatisfaction among nurses. This unhealthy situation contributes to nurses leaving their positions and often their profession altogether. More than half of nurses surveyed report they have been subject to verbal abuse and over 90% have witnessed disruptive behavior. Nurses can encounter conflict in every dimension of their work. Be it conflict with others, or between their own personal and professional values, skilled communication supports the ethical obligation to seek resolution that preserves a nurse's professional integrity while ensuring a patient's safety and best interests.

Ensuring that nurses are provided the education, competency mastery and rewards to effectively negotiate these conflict-laden conditions would itself dramatically alter the environment.

Critical Elements

- The health care organization provides team members with support for and access to education programs that develop critical communication skills including self-awareness, inquiry/dialogue, conflict management, negotiation, advocacy and listening.
- Skilled communicators focus on finding solutions and achieving desirable outcomes.
- Skilled communicators seek to protect and advance collaborative relationships among colleagues.
- Skilled communicators invite and hear all relevant perspectives.
- Skilled communicators call upon goodwill and mutual respect to build consensus and arrive at common understanding.
- Skilled communicators demonstrate congruence between words and actions, holding others accountable for doing the same.
- The health care organization establishes zero-tolerance policies and enforces them to address and eliminate abuse and disrespectful behavior in the workplace.
- The health care organization establishes formal structures and processes that ensure effective information sharing among patients, families and the health care team.
- Skilled communicators have access to appropriate communication technologies and are proficient in their use.
- The health care organization establishes systems that require individuals and teams to formally evaluate the impact of communication on clinical, financial and work environment outcomes.

- The health care organization includes communication as a criterion in its formal performance appraisal system and team members demonstrate skilled communication to qualify for professional advancement.

Standard 2: True Collaboration

Nurses must be relentless in pursuing and fostering true collaboration.

True collaboration is a process, not an event. It must be ongoing and build over time, eventually resulting in a work culture where joint communication and decision making between nurses and other disciplines and among nurses themselves becomes the norm. Unlike the lip service that collaboration is often given, in true collaboration the unique knowledge and abilities of each professional are respected to achieve safe, quality care for patients. Skilled communication, trust, knowledge, shared responsibility, mutual respect, optimism and coordination are integral to successful collaboration.

Without the synchronous, ongoing collaborative work of health care professionals from multiple disciplines, patient and family needs cannot be optimally satisfied within the complexities of today's health care system. Extensive evidence shows the negative impact of poor collaboration on various measurable indicators including patient and family satisfaction, patient safety and outcomes, professional staff satisfaction, nurse retention and cost. The Institute of Medicine points to "a historical lack of interprofessional cooperation" as one of the cultural barriers to safety in hospitals.

Nearly 90% of the American Association of Critical-Care Nurses' members and constituents report that collaboration with physicians and administrators is among the most important elements in creating a healthy work environment. Further, nurse–physician collaboration has been found to be one of the three strongest predictors of psychological empowerment of nurses. Mutual respect between nurses and physicians for each other's knowledge and competence, coupled with a mutual concern that quality patient care will be provided are key organizational elements of work environments that attract and retain nurses. Additionally, an unresponsive bureaucracy generates organizational stress, which is significantly more predictive of nurse burnout and resignations than emotional stressors inherent in the work itself.

Collaboration requires constant attention and nurturing, supported by formal processes and structures that foster joint communication and decision making. Evidence documenting differing perceptions about the importance and effectiveness of nurse–physician collaboration among nurses, physicians and health care executives points to an imperative that effective methods be developed to improve working relationships between nurses and physicians.

Critical Elements

- The health care organization provides team members with support for and access to education programs that develop collaboration skills.
- The health care organization creates, uses and evaluates processes that define each team member's accountability for collaboration and how unwillingness to collaborate will be addressed.
- The health care organization creates, uses and evaluates operational structures that ensure the decision making authority of nurses is acknowledged and incorporated as the norm.
- The health care organization ensures unrestricted access to structured forums, such as ethics committees, and makes available the time needed to resolve disputes among all critical participants, including patients, families and the health care team.
- Every team member embraces true collaboration as an ongoing process and invests in its development to ensure a sustained culture of collaboration.
- Every team member contributes to the achievement of common goals by giving power and respect to each person's voice, integrating individual differences, resolving competing interests and safeguarding the essential contribution each must make in order to achieve optimal outcomes.
- Every team member acts with a high level of personal integrity.
- Team members master skilled communication, an essential element of true collaboration.
- Each team member demonstrates competence appropriate to his or her role and responsibilities.
- Nurse managers and medical directors are equal partners in modeling and fostering true collaboration.

Standard 3: Effective Decision Making

Nurses must be valued and committed partners in making policy, directing and evaluating clinical care and leading organizational operations.

In order to fulfill their role as advocates, nurses must be involved in making decisions about patient care. A significant gap often

exists between what nurses are accountable for and their ability to participate in decisions that affect those accountabilities. Evidence suggests that physicians, pharmacists, administrators and nurses assign primary responsibility for patient safety to nurses. However, only 8% of physicians recognize nurses as part of the decision making team. Other research reports that a majority of nurses feel relatively powerless to change things they dislike in their work environment. This autonomy accountability gap interferes with nurses' ability to optimize their essential contribution and fulfill their obligations to the public as licensed professionals.

As the single constant professional presence with hospitalized patients, nurses uniquely gather, filter, interpret and transform data from patients and the system into the meaningful information required to diagnose, treat and deliver care to a patient. This data management role of nurses is a vital link in the decision making activities of the entire health care team. Failure to incorporate the experienced perspective of nurses in clinical and operational decisions may result in costly errors, jeopardize patient safety and threaten the financial viability of health care organizations.

Nurses believe that they provide high-quality nursing care and are accountable for their own practice. Nurses who do not have control over their practice become dissatisfied and are at risk for leaving an organization. Health care organizations recognized for attracting and retaining nurses have successfully implemented professional care models in which nurses have the responsibility and related authority for patient care along with formal operational structures that support autonomous nursing practice. Their success is recognized by national programs such as the AACN Beacon Award for Critical Care Excellence, the Magnet Nursing Services Recognition Program and the Baldrige National Quality Program.

Critical Elements

- The health care organization provides team members with support for and access to ongoing education and development programs focusing on strategies that assure collaborative decision making. Program content includes mutual goal setting, negotiation, facilitation, conflict management, systems thinking and performance improvement.
- The health care organization clearly articulates organizational values and team members incorporate these values when making decisions.
- The health care organization has operational structures in place that ensure the perspectives of patients and their

families are incorporated into every decision affecting patient care.

- Individual team members share accountability for effective decision making by acquiring necessary skills, mastering relevant content, assessing situations accurately, sharing fact-based information, communicating professional opinions clearly and inquiring actively.
- The health care organization establishes systems, such as structured forums involving all departments and health care disciplines, to facilitate data-driven decisions.
- The health care organization establishes deliberate decision making processes that ensure respect for the rights of every individual, incorporate all key perspectives and designate clear accountability.
- The health care organization has fair and effective processes in place at all levels to objectively evaluate the results of decisions, including delayed decisions and indecision.

Standard 4: Appropriate Staffing

Staffing must ensure the effective match between patient needs and nurse competencies.

Inappropriate staffing is one of the most harmful threats to patient safety and to the well-being of nurses. Evidence suggests that better patient outcomes result when a higher proportion of care hours is provided by registered nurses, as compared with care by licensed practical nurses or nursing assistants. The likelihood of death or serious complications after surgery increases when fewer nurses are assigned to care for patients. Further research supports a relationship between specialty certification and clinical nursing expertise.

Because nurses intercept 86% of all medication errors made by other professionals, an increase in these errors will likely occur when nurses are overworked, overstressed and in short supply. Inadequate staffing leads to nurse dissatisfaction, burnout and turnover. Nurse turnover jeopardizes the quality of care, increases patient costs and decreases hospital profitability. Staffing is a complex process with the goal of matching the needs of patients at multiple points throughout their illness with the skills and competencies of nurses. Because the condition of critically ill patients rapidly and continuously fluctuates, flexibility of nurse staffing that goes beyond fixed nurse-to-patient ratios is imperative. Relying on staffing ratios alone ignores variance in patient needs and acuity.

Organizations must engage in dramatic innovation to devise and systematically test new staffing models. All staffing models require methods for ongoing evaluation of staffing decisions in relation to patient and system outcomes. This evaluation is essential in order to provide accurate trend data from which targeted improvement tactics—including technologies to reduce the demand and increase the efficiency of nurses' work—can be undertaken.

Critical Elements

- The health care organization has staffing policies in place that are solidly grounded in ethical principles and support the professional obligation of nurses to provide high quality care.
- Nurses participate in all organizational phases of the staffing process from education and planning—including matching nurses' competencies with patients' assessed needs—through evaluation.
- The health care organization has formal processes in place to evaluate the effect of staffing decisions on patient and system outcomes. This evaluation includes analysis of when patient needs and nurse competencies are mismatched and how often contingency plans are implemented.
- The health care organization has a system in place that facilitates team members' use of staffing and outcomes data to develop more effective staffing models.
- The health care organization provides support services at every level of activity to ensure nurses can optimally focus on the priorities and requirements of patient and family care.
- The health care organization adopts technologies that increase the effectiveness of nursing care delivery. Nurses are engaged in the selection, adaptation and evaluation of these technologies.

Standard 5: Meaningful Recognition

Nurses must be recognized and must recognize others for the value each brings to the work of the organization.

Recognition of the value and meaningfulness of one's contribution to an organization's work is a fundamental human need and an essential requisite to personal and professional development. People who are not recognized feel invisible, undervalued, unmotivated and disrespected. A majority of nurses are dissatisfied with the recognition they receive from their employer. This lack of recognition leads to discontent, poor morale, reduced productivity and suboptimal care outcomes. Inadequate recognition is cited as a primary reason for turnover among employees and is linked to decreasing nurse satisfaction.

Three out of four American Association of Critical-Care Nurses' members and constituents rank recognition for their contributions as a central element of a healthy work environment. Hospitals recognized for attracting and retaining nurses emphasize personal growth and development, and provide multiple rewards for expertise and opportunities for clinical advancement.

Like true collaboration, meaningful recognition is a process, not an event. It must be ongoing and build over time, becoming a norm within the work culture. Recognition has meaning only when it is relevant to the person being recognized. Recognition that is not congruent with a person's contributions or comes in tandem with emotionally charged organizational change is often perceived as disrespectful tokenism. Effective programs of recognition will not occur automatically and require formal structures and processes to ensure desired outcomes.

Critical Elements

- The health care organization has a comprehensive system in place that includes formal processes and structured forums that ensure a sustainable focus on recognizing all team members for their contributions and the value they bring to the work of the organization.
- The health care organization establishes a systematic process for all team members to learn about the institution's recognition system and how to participate by recognizing the contributions of colleagues and the value they bring to the organization.
- The health care organization's recognition system reaches from the bedside to the board table, ensuring individuals receive recognition consistent with their personal definition of meaning, fulfillment, development and advancement at every stage of their professional career.
- The health care organization's recognition system includes processes which validate that recognition is meaningful to those being acknowledged.
- Team members understand that everyone is responsible for playing an active role in the organization's recognition program and meaningfully recognizing contributions.
- The health care organization regularly and comprehensively evaluates its recognition system, ensuring effective programs that help to move the organization toward a sustainable culture of excellence that values meaningful recognition.

Standard 6: Authentic Leadership

Nurse leaders must fully embrace the imperative of a healthy work environment, authentically live it and engage others in its achievement.

Less than half of the American Association of Critical-Care Nurses' members rank their relationships with their managers and administrators as positive, yet more than 90% identify effective leaders as an important element of a healthy work environment. A multitude of reports and white papers issued by leaders in all sectors of the health care community document the issue of inadequately positioned and prepared leaders in nursing and strongly call for effective measures to strengthen nursing leadership.

Nurse leaders—including managers, administrators, advanced practice nurses, educators and other formal and informal clinical leaders—seldom have the support resources commensurate with their scope of responsibilities and often do not have access to key decision making forums within health care organizations. Nurse managers in particular are key to the retention of satisfied staff yet, all too often, receive little preparation, education, coaching or mentoring to ensure success in their role. Nurse leaders must be skilled communicators, team builders, agents for positive change, committed to service, results oriented and role models for collaborative practice. This requires skill in the core competencies of self-knowledge, strategic vision, risk-taking and creativity, interpersonal and communication effectiveness, and inspiration.

Healthy work environments require that individual nurses and organizations commit to the development of nurse leaders in a systematic and comprehensive way. Nurse leaders must be positioned within key operational and governance bodies of the organization in order to inform and influence decisions that affect nursing practice and the environment in which it is practiced.

Critical Elements

- The health care organization provides support for and access to educational programs to ensure that nurse leaders develop and enhance knowledge and abilities in: skilled communication, effective decision making, true collaboration, meaningful recognition, and ensuring resources to achieve appropriate staffing.
- Nurse leaders demonstrate an understanding of the requirements and dynamics at the point of care and within this context successfully translate the vision of a healthy work environment.

- Nurse leaders excel at generating visible enthusiasm for achieving the standards that create and sustain healthy work environments.
- Nurse leaders lead the design of systems necessary to effectively implement and sustain standards for healthy work environments.
- The health care organization ensures that nurse leaders are appropriately positioned in their pivotal role in creating and sustaining healthy work environments. This includes participation in key decision making forums, access to essential information and the authority to make necessary decisions.
- The health care organization facilitates the efforts of nurse leaders to create and sustain a healthy work environment by providing the necessary time and financial and human resources.
- The health care organization provides a formal co-mentoring program for all nurse leaders. Nurse leaders actively engage in the co-mentoring program.
- Nurse leaders role model skilled communication, true collaboration, effective decision-making, meaningful recognition and authentic leadership.
- The health care organization includes the leadership contribution to creating and sustaining a healthy work environment as a criterion in each nurse leader's performance appraisal. Nurse leaders must demonstrate sustained leadership in creating and sustaining a healthy work environment to achieve professional advancement.
- Nurse leaders and team members mutually and objectively evaluate the impact of leadership processes and decisions on the organization's progress toward creating and sustaining a healthy work environment.

Call to Action

Healthy work environments are essential to ensure patient safety, enhance staff recruitment and retention, and maintain an organization's financial viability. Inattention to relationship issues poses a serious obstacle to creating and sustaining those environments. Without them, the journey to excellence is impossible.

The six standards put forth in this document offer the framework for health care organizations to elevate these competencies to the highest strategic and operational importance. The ensuing dialogue will guide the fundamental reprioritization and reallocation of resources necessary to create and sustain healthy work environments.

Visions of the Future

Health professionals in many organizations across the United States have begun their journey toward creating and sustaining healthy work environments. They have committed to addressing the tough issues that block the way. These powerful stories illuminate what is possible in work environments that call forth each individual's optimal contribution. Their inspiring successes paint a vivid picture of how this is necessary.

Listen. Learn. Act. The future of American health care depends on it.

Skilled communication protects and advances collaborative relationships.

The doctor has superb knowledge about medicine and I have superb knowledge about nursing. Because of my constant assessment and observation, I know how the patient is responding to his illness and treatment better than the doctor does. Furthermore, we need each other's knowledge if we're going to help a patient. We respect each other and don't have to tiptoe around about what we think and observe. Once, we worked together all night on a 3-pound baby with generalized sepsis. We continually discussed what studies said should be done and not done. We tried one thing, then another, but unfortunately the baby died. Yet even in her grief, the mother told us how impressed she was at how we worked together. She said she could see her baby was receiving the best care possible.

True collaboration is an ongoing process built on mutual trust and respect.

Doctors and nurses in our unit have a mutual trust and respect that's outstanding. Doctors value nurses' opinions. If we say, "You need to come," they do and know we are not overreacting. And it's not just me and one or two docs; it's all of them. We make sure that we don't lose this trust, this respect.

We are evaluated on how we work with the doctors. Do we work collaboratively? Do we put the patient first? And we make sure the new grads or even new hires talk to the doc "right." I teach new graduates that you don't call a doctor at three in the morning with a routine update that can wait.

You carefully assess the patient and you bring all your knowledge and skill to bear. So when you do have to call, the doctor knows she's really needed and will hustle to get here.

Nurse leaders create a vision for a healthy work environment and model it in all their actions.

Why did I come to work here? Because of the nurse manager. When she interviewed me, she asked me what kind of support I would need from her. The openness of her question impressed me, so I told her. She said she could meet my expectations. Not try to or maybe, but that she could. Our manager is so respectful of the nurses, of our knowledge and of what we do. Day after day, her words and actions show that she believes each of us is very valuable. At unit meetings, our manager is the one who reminds us that what nurses know is different, but just as important, as what doctors know. She has earned my trust and respect, and I know I have earned hers. That's why I'm here and why I'll stay.

Meaningful recognition acknowledges the value of a person's contribution to the work of the organization.

"He's stable and doing all right," the outgoing nurse said during last night's shift report. To the receiving nurse, the patient was more restless than she thought he should be. His face was taut, yet his vital signs had not changed. The nurse consulted other more experienced nurses. They agreed with her observations, advising her to call the physician if she continued to feel uneasy or uncomfortable, or if the patient's vital signs changed. At 2:00 A.M. the nurse called the physician to describe what she saw and felt, including her inability to substantiate it with changes in vital signs. She emphasized the need for the physician to come in. He did and immediately started treatment for a collapsed lung. The nurse felt she had gone out on a limb in calling, but said she had faith in her own judgment. "Good call," the physician complimented her this morning, as did several nurses and our nurse manager. The nurse said this was something she would remember the rest of her life.

Remaining focused on matching nurses' competencies to patients' needs points the way to innovative staffing solutions.

Yesterday was one of the craziest days I can remember in this ICU. Patients waiting to be transferred in. Emergency open-heart surgery in progress. A full Emergency Department. Like most days, our best-laid staffing plans looked hopeless. It was time to brainstorm at the assignment board. Our nurse manager and house supervisor joined us. Everyone's ideas were taken seriously and we came up with a new plan that really worked. An on-call nurse came in. Two orientees were reassigned so they could still learn, but help their preceptors more. One nurse took an extra patient until he was transferred. Each time a new patient arrived, we double-teamed until things settled down. Our manager stayed until we were sure the plan would work. At the end of the shift we were all tired, but proud that we developed a plan for our patients to get the best care. That's what teamwork means for me.

Advocating for patients requires involvement in decisions that affect patient care.

As a staff nurse, I never thought I would say this. I wouldn't miss our Product Evaluation Committee meeting. My manager asked me to be on the committee and I didn't even know what they did. Turns out they decide whether or not to buy certain products for the whole hospital—most of which affect nursing care. They listen to me when I talk about which products work for patients and which ones don't. Just the other day, the chairperson told me most committee members would never know a bedside nurse's perspective and thanked me again for the time I invest in the committee. I never knew my voice could make such a difference.[1]

Source: This appendix is a robust excerpt from the American Association of Critical Care Nurses' publication *Healthy Work Environments* and is reprinted here with permission.

Reference

1. These illustrations are adapted from interviews with nurses in Magnet hospitals obtained by Marlene F. Kramer and Claudia Schmalenberg during the Dimensions of Magnetism study. See also Chapter 2 of McClure M., Hinshaw A.S.: *Magnet Hospitals Revisited: Attraction and Retention of Professional Nurses.* Washington, DC: American Nurses Publishing, 2002.

Index